MOSBY'S®

Pathophysiology Memory NoteCards

Visual, Mnemonic, and Memory Aids for Nurses

THIRD EDITION

MOSBY'S®
Pathophysiology Memory NoteCards

Visual, Mnemonic, and Memory Aids for Nurses

JULIA L. ROGERS, DNP, APRN, CNS, FNP-BC, FAANP
Assistant Professor
Purdue University Northwest
Hammond, Indiana;
Nurse Practitioner
Northwest Health Medical Group: Pulmonary and Critical Care
Valparaiso, Indiana

John Quinn, Illustrator

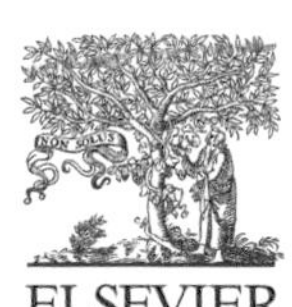

ELSEVIER

ELSEVIER
3251 Riverport Lane
St. Louis, Missouri 63043

MOSBY'S® PATHOPHYSIOLOGY MEMORY NOTECARDS, THIRD EDITION

ISBN: 978-0-323-83229-8

Content Strategist: Heather Bays-Petrovic
Senior Content Development Specialist: Rebecca Leenhouts
Director, Content Development: Laurie Gower
Publishing Services Manager: Deepthi Unni
Senior Project Manager: Umarani Natarajan
Design Direction: Brian Salisbury

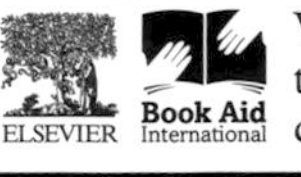

Printed in India

Last digit is the print number: 9 8 7 6 5 4 3 2 1

Contents

BODY'S SELF-DEFENSE

CELLULAR PROLIFERATION

PULMONARY SYSTEM

CARDIOVASCULAR SYSTEM

HEMATOLOGIC SYSTEM

ENDOCRINE SYSTEM

MUSCULOSKELETAL SYSTEM

SENSORY SYSTEM

NERVOUS SYSTEM

GASTROINTESTINAL SYSTEM

HEPATIC AND BILIARY SYSTEMS

RENAL AND UROLOGIC SYSTEM

REPRODUCTIVE SYSTEM

INTEGUMENTARY SYSTEM

Dedication

Dedicated to all my past, present, and future pathophysiology students. Thanks for being inquisitive and wanting to learn about the human body's disordered physiological processes that cause disease. This is also dedicated to all the lives lost to SARS Co-V-2 (COVID-19) and to their families.

—Julia L. Rogers

Special thanks to my wife, Diana, who has always been there for me and my art.

—John Quinn

Acknowledgments

I want to take the time to acknowledge some of the individuals and teams that provided so much support and time in this project.

First, thanks to the amazing illustrator, John Quinn. He was able to see the vision of what was needed to help students learn through art. You are an amazing artist and I hope we continue to work together in future endeavors.

A special thanks to senior production manager Urmarani Natarajan, for always making sure everything was in order. You were a wonderful part of the project which could not have been completed without your assistance. I am grateful to have had you on this team.

The entire production team deserves acknowledgment Heather, Laurie, Rebecca, Deepthi, Urmarani, and Brian. It is because of the entire team and all the working parts that this project has been completed. Thank you for all you have contributed, I appreciate each one of you.

Thanks to Heather Bays-Petrovic, Laurie Gower, and Tamara Myers for believing in me and John to take on the project.

A big thanks to my family, Dwayne, Zachery, and Shane that always provide me with the space and time needed for my writing projects. I appreciate all of you more than you will ever know.

Finally, thanks to my biggest fans and support system—Vesta, Jeannie, Joni, Doug, Letty, Lucy, and Dionne. You have all hung in there with me and remained my rocks.

IMMUNE SYSTEM

The immune system is a complex system of cells and proteins that fight and defend the body against invasion of unwanted foreign substances. There are two layers including the innate (non-specific) and the adaptive (specific) immune systems.

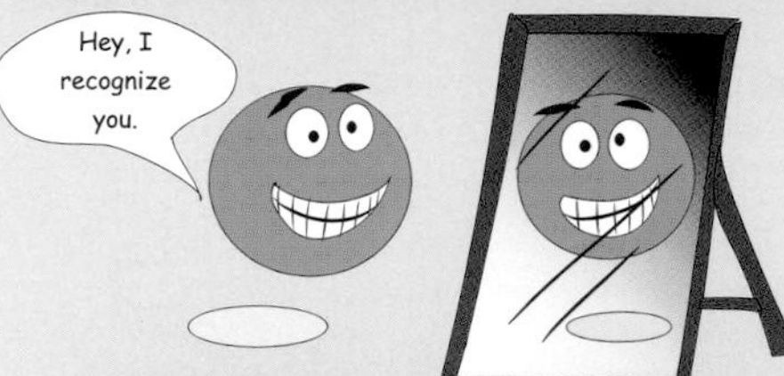

The immune system can be activated by foreign substances called antigens, which include infectious agents, environmental substances, and cancer.

The body recognizes itself and foreign antigens with the help of an identification tag.

Sometimes the immune system identifies itself as foreign and attacks.

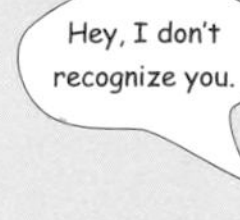

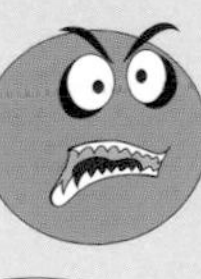

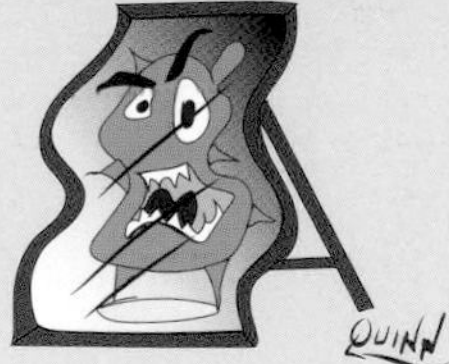

What You Need to Know

Immune System

SIGNIFICANCE OF THE IMMUNE SYSTEM

Immunity protects the body from invading toxic substances and infectious microorganisms. A competent immune system will prevent diseases when the body is exposed. Immunity involves an antigen–antibody response to protect the body against invading organisms.

TYPES OF IMMUNITY

- **Innate (natural) immunity**—is present at birth and protects the body against diseases.
- **Acquired immunity**—is gained after birth.
  - *Active immunity:*
    - Natural—exposure to infectious pathogen, develops disease, and creates antibodies against pathogen (chickenpox, measles, hepatitis).
    - Artificial—immunizations are administered to create antibodies.
  - *Passive immunity:*
    - Natural—infant receives it from the mother at birth.
    - Artificial—preformed antibodies (immunoglobulins) are injected. The antibodies are short lived because the body does not produce its own.

SELF-RECOGNITION

Each cell has a unique "product code," which allows the immune system to recognize its own body cells and allows for the "self versus nonself" recognition of cells. This ability is critical to prevent the immune system from attacking the normal healthy cells of the body.

SOURCES OF ANTIGENS

- Infectious—bacteria, viruses, fungi, parasites
- Noninfectious—pollen, vaccines, organ transplants, blood transfusions

HOMEOSTASIS

The body maintains homeostasis with built-in defenses that protect against invading organisms.

- Physical, mechanical, or biochemical barriers.
- Leukocytes destroy invading microorganisms by a process known as *phagocytosis* and *enzyme digestion.*

- The spleen works to remove damaged and old cells to maintain a healthy balance.
- Inflammatory response—occurs after cellular or tissue injury.

NURSING MANAGEMENT

- Patients who are chronically ill are at a high risk for impaired immune response.
- Hand hygiene is the single most important factor for the prevention of infection.
- Educate the patient on the importance of handwashing.
- Encourage the patient to maintain current immunizations.

Important nursing implications
Serious/life-threatening implications
Most frequent side effects
Patient teaching

INNATE IMMUNITY

Innate immunity is nonspecific and is the body's defense system that you have since birth.

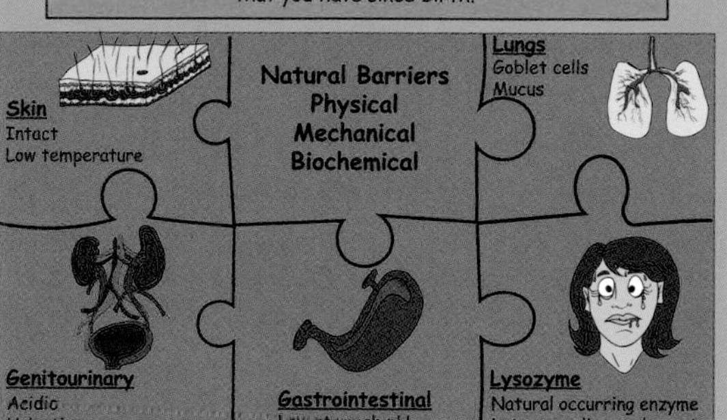

Dendritic cell
Mast cell
T cell
Macrophage
Natural killer cell
Basophil
Natural killer T cell
Complement protein
Neutrophil
Eosinophil

Quinn

The innate immune system is mediated by granulocytes, mast cells, dendritic cells, macrophages, and NK cells. Complement proteins are also part of the first line of defense against infection.

What You Need to Know

Innate Immunity

SIGNIFICANCE OF INNATE IMMUNITY

Innate immunity is the first line of defense against invading pathogens. Innate immunity is the body's defense system that is present at birth. Innate immunity is nonspecific, meaning anything that is identified as foreign or nonself is a target for the innate immune response.

INNATE IMMUNE RESPONSE

The innate immune response consists of physical, chemical, and biochemical barriers.

- Physical barriers: Skin, membranous lining of the gastrointestinal (GI), respiratory, and urinary tracts.
- Mechanical barriers: Vomiting, micturition, low skin temperature, and low pH of the stomach.
- Biochemical barriers: Mucus, saliva, perspiration, tears, and earwax.
- The innate immune system is mediated by several types of white blood cells or leukocytes, which work to defend the body against foreign toxins known as antigens. The following cells are important defenders: granulocytes, mast cells, macrophages, dendritic cells, and natural killer (NK) cells.
- The complement cascade plays a major role in the innate immune system and may directly destroy pathogens, but it also works with and supports the components of the inflammatory response. Proteins of the complement system are some of the strongest agents against bacteria.
- Inflammation is the second line defense of the innate immune system. Inflammation occurs as a response to chemical signals that are responding to microbial infection and/or tissue damage. The inflammatory process is part of innate and adaptive immune systems.

Antigens stimulate the immune system response. The body recognizes antigens as foreign to the body, and the immune response begins to produce antibodies against specific antigens.

Important nursing implications | Serious/life-threatening implications
Most frequent side effects | Patient teaching

ADAPTIVE IMMUNITY

The adaptive immune system makes antibodies to fight specific antigens that it has previously encountered and stored in its memory. The B cells and T cells are the main responders to a stimulus.

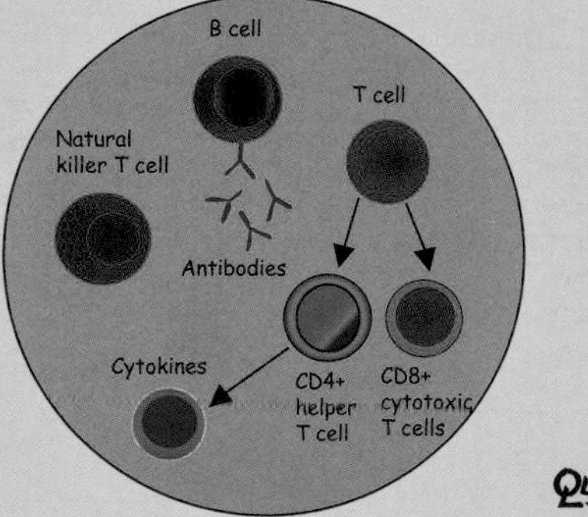

Once the T helper cell recognizes a foreign substance, they alert the B cell to divide and form clones, which produce specific antibodies to fight the antigen. Some of the B cell clones are plasma cells that produce antibodies and march into battle. Other B cell clones become memory cells, providing long term immunity.

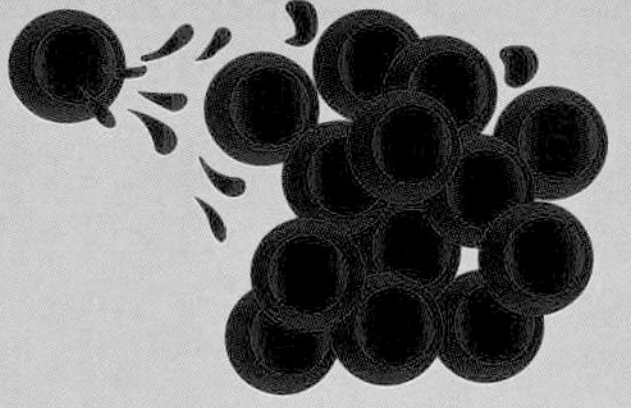

What You Need to Know

Adaptive Immunity

SIGNIFICANCE OF ADAPTIVE IMMUNITY

Adaptive immunity occurs naturally from exposure to a pathogen or vaccination. The body produces antibodies with the initial disease and the presence of antibodies prevents a recurrence of the disease. The adaptive immune system is activated when the innate immune system is insufficient to control an infection. The adaptive immune system is antigen and antibody specific and involves memory to provide the host with long-term protection from reinfection.

Types of adaptive response: Immunity occurs as a result of the invasion of foreign protein (antigen) and is the result of many different cells working together throughout the body to recognize another invasion of the same antigen.

- **Cell-mediated immunity**—assists in regulating the process of the inflammatory response and the interactions of the T lymphocytes supporting the antibody-mediated process of immunity.
- **Humoral immunity (antibody-mediated immunity)**—invasion by a foreign protein or antigen will initiate the production of antibodies by the B cells. B cells form memory cells and are produced to allow for future recognition of the antigen.

ADAPTIVE IMMUNE RESPONSE

The body produces B and T lymphocyte cells when it recognizes a foreign antigen in the body, which initiates the body's immune response. Antibodies are formed against the foreign agent (antigen).

- **B cells**—are lymphocytes that are developed to be specific to only one antigen. Antigen recognition, antibody production, and development of memory cells or sustained immunity are provided. *B cells* secrete antibodies that are specific to the antigen and will attach to it.
  - *Memory B cells*—recognize antigens from memory and attack it if the antigen invades again.
  - *Antibodies*—neutralize the toxins and viruses and assist in destroying the bacteria, as well as activate the inflammatory response.
- **T cells**—are also lymphocytes that attack the antigen. Several types of *T cells* exist, and each performs a different function:
  - *Cytotoxic T cells*—release toxic substances to kill certain antigens.
  - *Memory T cells*—recognize the antigen and prevent it from invading the body by using antibodies that were previously produced to target the antigen.
  - *Helper T cells*—help balance and control the cell-mediated response.

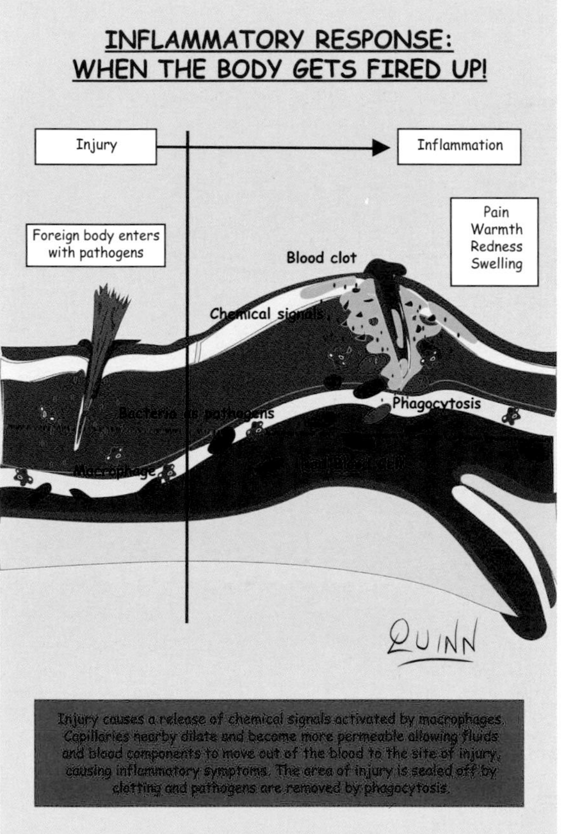
INFLAMMATORY RESPONSE:
WHEN THE BODY GETS FIRED UP!
Injury
Inflammation
Foreign body enters with pathogens
Pain
Warmth
Redness
Swelling
Blood clot
Chemical signals
Phagocytosis
Bacteria as pathogens
Macrophage
QUINN
Injury causes a release of chemical signals activated by macrophages. Capillaries nearby dilate and become more permeable allowing fluids and blood components to move out of the blood to the site of injury, causing inflammatory symptoms. The area of injury is sealed off by clotting and pathogens are removed by phagocytosis.

What You Need to Know

Inflammatory Response

SIGNIFICANCE OF INFLAMMATION

Immunity works with inflammation to protect the body from both injury and invading microorganisms. Inflammation occurs rapidly as a response to cell injury, but does not provide immunity or protection against the invasion of future organisms. Inflammation is not the same as *infection*. Inflammation occurs without infection, but inflammation most often occurs with infection. Inflammation develops as a result of an injury to the cell by infectious (bacteria) or noninfectious (injury) agents.

SIGNS AND SYMPTOMS

- Redness, swelling, heat, pain, and loss of function.

VASCULAR RESPONSE IN INFLAMMATION

Histamines, prostaglandins, and kinins are released when cell damage occurs. Vasodilation occurs with increased vascular permeability, which leads to increased blood flow to the site of the injury. This action is responsible for the signs and symptoms of inflammation.

CELLULAR RESPONSE IN INFLAMMATION

After cell injury occurs, WBCs (neutrophils and monocytes) travel to the injured site to clean up the area before healing can occur. Neutrophils arrive first and engulf the damaged cells and other bacteria. Because of their short life span (6–12 hours), neutrophils quickly die and develop into *exudate* or *pus*. Monocytes and macrophages travel to the site in 3–7 days and clean the injured site. Lymphocytes also travel to the site, initiating the immune response. Basophils aid in the process by releasing histamine. After an allergic reaction (e.g., beesting), eosinophils travel to the injured site.

INFLAMMATION AND REPAIR

Inflammation

- Destroys the agent that caused the injury; removes it from the site.
- Walls off and confines the agent to limit the effects of the damage.
- Stimulates and enhances the immune response; promotes healing.
- Inflammation is nonspecific. Unlike the immune response, inflammation occurs in the same manner with each exposure, regardless of the causative agent.

HIV AND CORONAVIRUS IN CHILDREN AND INFANTS

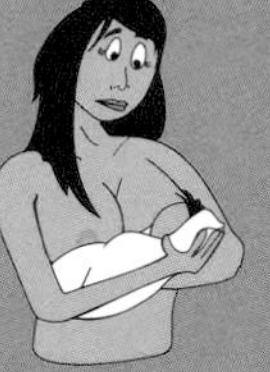

HIV can be transmitted across the placenta or by contact with infected blood/secretions at birth, and through breast milk.

Multisystem inflammatory syndrome in children (MIS-C) is a condition that may inflame different organs of the body. Many children with MIS-C had the virus that causes COVID-19. In COVID-19 a rash may present in children and infants.

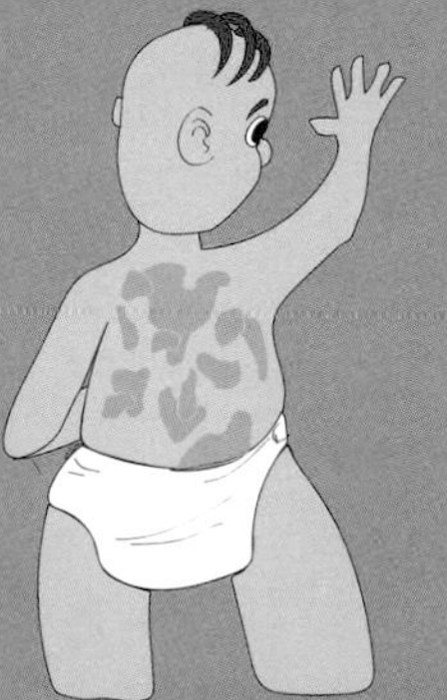

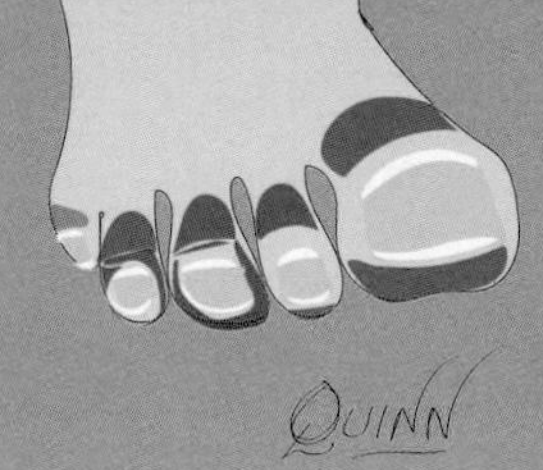

Young children who test positive for coronavirus may develop swelling and discoloration on one or several toes or fingers, known as "COVID toes."

QUINN

What You Need to Know

HIV and Coronavirus in Children and Infants

SIGNIFICANCE OF THE HUMAN IMMUNODEFICIENCY VIRUS

The human immunodeficiency virus (HIV) attacks the DNA of the CD4-T cells and makes the cells weak and ineffective components of the immune system. Everyone who has acquired immunodeficiency syndrome (AIDS) is positive for HIV; however, everyone who is positive for HIV does not necessarily have AIDS.

SIGNIFICANCE OF CORONAVIRUS

Coronavirus (SARS-CoV-2) has the potential to cause multisystem inflammatory syndrome in children (MIS-C), which is a condition that causes acute organ inflammation. Infants (age <1 year) and children with underlying medical conditions might be at increased risk for severe illness from SARS-CoV-2 infection. The incubation period of SARS-CoV-2 for children is 2–14 days with an average of 6 days.

TRANSMISSION IN CHILDREN

- **HIV** Transmission is significantly reduced if the mother has been treated with antiretroviral medications during pregnancy.
  - Perinatal transmission—accounts for over 90% of transmissions in children. Exposure to infected blood and secretions during birth; transplacental exposure in utero; breast feeding—transmission occurs after delivery.
- **SARS-CoV-2**
  - Transmission is person to person by airborne small droplets and particles that contain virus landing on the eyes, nose, or mouth.

DIAGNOSIS

- **HIV**
  - Because the infant receives maternal antibodies, it complicates the process of identifying the antibodies in the newborn. Infants can usually be diagnosed by 1 month of age depending on the viral load. Newborns of HIV-positive mothers should be screened at 24 hours, at 1–2 months, and at 3–6 months. A positive test should be confirmed by a second test.
  - Approximately 30% of infants infected with HIV at birth will become symptomatic within the first 2 years.
- **SARS-CoV-2**
  - PCR test is the standard for diagnosis in symptomatic or asymptomatic children with SARS-CoV-2 exposure.

- Many children are asymptomatic, but may have fever, cough, shortness of breath, fatigue, loss of taste or smell, headache, muscle and joint pain, nausea, vomiting, or diarrhea.
- A blotchy rash on the skin is often times present in children with SARS-CoV-2, but can be present with other viruses. The rash may appear as red areas on the toes of children that gradually turn purple. It is sometimes called "COVID toes."

NURSING IMPLICATION

- Most common opportunistic infection in HIV and SARS-CoV-2 is pneumonia.
- *Pneumocystis jirovecii* pneumonia (also known as pneumocystic pneumonia [PCP]) is the most common pneumonia in HIV. All infants of HIV-positive mothers should receive prophylaxis from birth.
- HIV positive infants and children fail to thrive and have nutritional deficiencies. Progressive encephalopathy is indicative of a poor prognosis.
- Children should be vaccinated and parents educated on the importance of vaccinations.

Important nursing implications	Serious/life-threatening implications
Most frequent side effects	Patient teaching

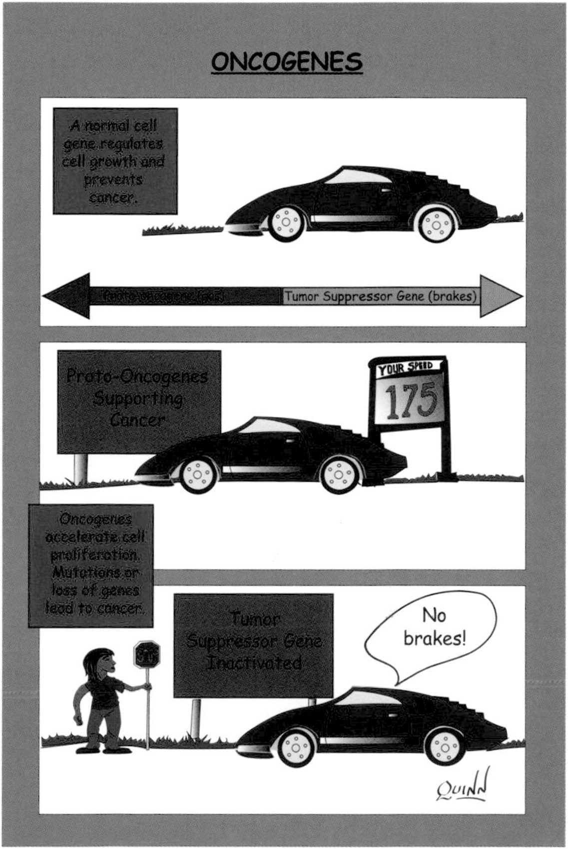

ONCOGENES

A normal cell gene regulates cell growth and prevents cancer.

Proto-oncogene (gas)

Tumor Suppressor Gene (brakes)

Proto-Oncogenes Supporting Cancer

YOUR SPEED

175

Oncogenes accelerate cell proliferation. Mutations or loss of genes lead to cancer.

Tumor Suppressor Gene Inactivated

No brakes!

QUINN

What You Need to Know

Oncogenes

CELLULAR DIFFERENTIATION

An orderly process where unspecialized cells progress from an immature state to a mature and specialized state.

SIGNIFICANCE OF ONCOGENES

- Oncogenes are mutant genes that have a dominant effect because only one of the cell's two gene copies has mutated. This mutation is a key feature of oncogene activity because a single altered gene copy leads to unregulated growth with the potential to transform a cell into a tumor cell. Oncogenes result from the *activation* of proto-oncogenes. These genes are in contrast to tumor suppressor genes, which must BOTH be defective to lead to abnormal cell division. Tumor suppressor genes cause cancer when they are *inactivated.*
- Normal genes that can be affected by mutation are the following two types:
  - *Proto-oncogenes*—genes that regulate cell growth. Mutations activate proto-oncogenes to function as oncogenes (tumor-producing genes) causing the cell to grow and divide at an accelerated out of control rate, which can lead to cancer.
  - *Tumor-suppressor genes*—suppress tumor cell growth and cell division, repair DNA errors, and support apoptosis. When mutated, tumor-suppressor genes become inactive, losing tumor suppression ability, which allows uncontrolled cell division and tumor growth.
- In addition to ordinary mutation, there is also *tumor virus*:
  - Viruses shed from tumors that infect normal growing cells by inserting the viral RNA or DNA into the normal cell, which may transform the normal cells into tumor cells.

EXAMPLES OF TUMOR SUPPRESSOR GENES

- Breast cancer (BRCA1/BRCA2)
- Retinoblastoma (RB1)
- Familial melanoma (CDKN2A)
- Neurofibromatosis (NF1)

Important nursing implications	Serious/life-threatening implications
Most frequent side effects	Patient teaching

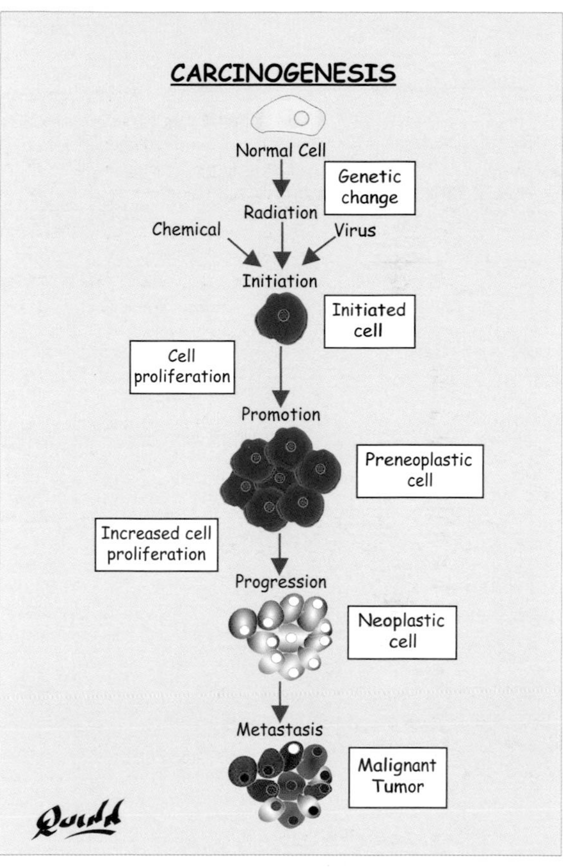
CARCINOGENESIS
Normal Cell
Genetic change
Radiation
Chemical
Virus
Initiation
Initiated cell
Cell proliferation
Promotion
Preneoplastic cell
Increased cell proliferation
Progression
Neoplastic cell
Metastasis
Malignant Tumor

What You Need to Know

Carcinogenesis—Process of Tumor Development

SIGNIFICANCE OF CARCINOGENESIS

Carcinogenesis is a multistep process that begins with the development of genotoxic (DNA toxic) changes within the normal cell. The cell can no longer control its own growth or location. It will travel to distant tissues and colonize (metastasize) in those tissues.

THREE PHASES OF TUMOR DEVELOPMENT

1. **Initiation**—mutation of cell's genetic structure, resulting from an inherited mutation, an error during DNA replication, or after exposure to a carcinogen (cancer-causing agent capable of producing cellular alterations).
2. **Promotion**—occurs with additional changes to the cells, resulting in further genetic damage that eventually leads to proliferation and a *malignant conversion*. Prevention activities are focused on this stage to reduce the promoting factors of cancer (i.e., cigarette smoking, dietary fat, obesity, alcohol consumption, severe stress).
3. **Progression**—cells are increasingly malignant in appearance and behavior and develop into invasive cancer with metastases to distant body parts.

CANCER CELL CHARACTERISTICS

- Local increase in cell numbers
- Loss of normal arrangement of cells
- Cell shape and size vary from normal
- Division in an uncoordinated manner
- Destruction of neighboring tissue

TUMOR CELL MARKERS

Biologic markers associated with cancer cells may be found in the blood, spinal fluid, urine, or on the tumor membrane. Markers aid in:

- Screening and identifying individuals at increased risk for developing cancer.
- Diagnosing the specific type of tumor present.
- Monitoring the clinical course of the cancer, and assisting in determining the individual's response to treatment.

Important nursing implications	Serious/life-threatening implications
Most frequent side effects	Patient teaching

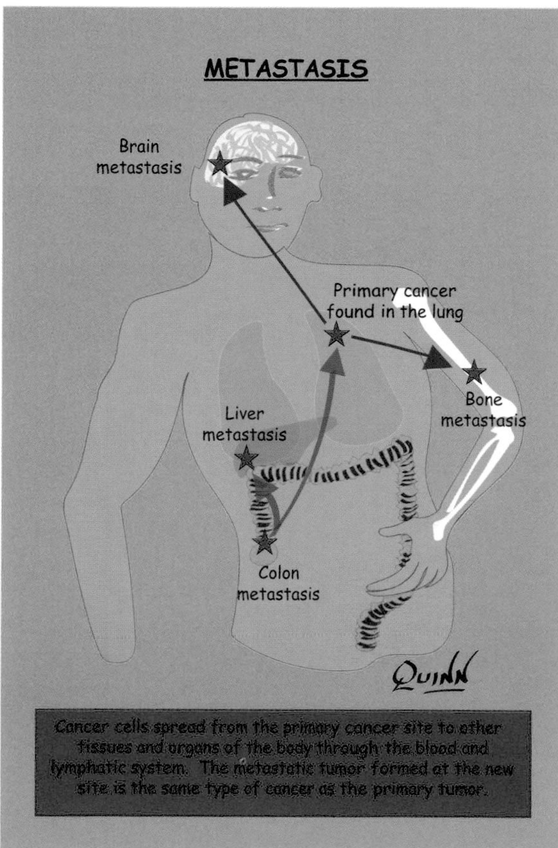
METASTASIS
Brain metastasis
Primary cancer found in the lung
Bone metastasis
Liver metastasis
Colon metastasis
QUINN
Cancer cells spread from the primary cancer site to other tissues and organs of the body through the blood and lymphatic system. The metastatic tumor formed at the new site is the same type of cancer as the primary tumor.

What You Need to Know

Metastasis

SIGNIFICANCE OF METASTASIS

Metastasis is the migration of cancer cells from the primary site or tumor where they originated to a distant site and the invasion of other tissues.

TUMOR SPREAD

Extension of the Primary Tumor Into Surrounding Areas

Tumors may spread to adjacent organs early in their development. This first step of the metastatic process most often occurs by direct extension of the tumor. As the tumor progresses, cells separate from the tumor and begin to invade the interstitial tissues. The spread of cancer cells also occurs secondary to the direct pressure of the tumor against the adjacent organ.

Metastasis Via Lymph and Veins

Malignant cells penetrate the blood vessels and lymphatic system. Cells are released and transported to a secondary site where they begin to proliferate. Cells also penetrate the body cavities. The most common route for distant metastasis is through the lymphatic system.

Angiogenesis

The growth of new blood vessels feed the tumor. The rate of the spread and growth of the tumor is directly related to the vascularity of the tumor. It must have adequate blood supply for oxygenation and nutrients, as well as growth cells to stimulate the growth of the tumor.

Metastatic Potential

Cancer cells grow and develop more rapidly when a vascular network has developed. However, a theory suggests that cancer cells, when stressed by hypoxia and poor nutrition, may actually survive to become the strongest and most aggressive cells of the tumor.

Distribution of Metastasis

Metastasis occurs by the cancer cells growing directly into the tissue surrounding the tumor, traveling in the blood, or traveling through the lymph system to nearby or distant locations. Some types of cancer show a preference to metastasize to certain organs. For example, kidney carcinomas often spread to bone and the thyroid. Some cancer cells are organ specific; they discriminate among different vascular beds and seek out certain other organs.

Important nursing implications | Serious/life-threatening implications

Most frequent side effects | Patient teaching

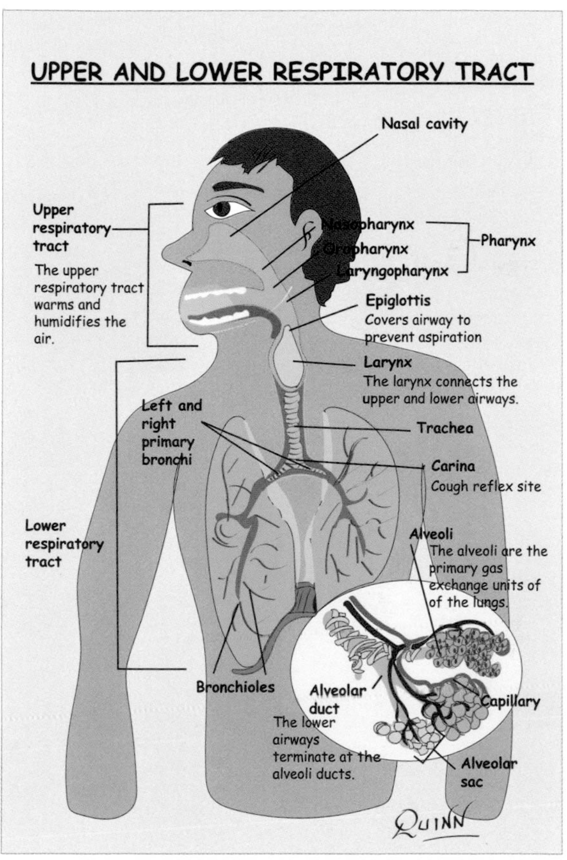
UPPER AND LOWER RESPIRATORY TRACT
Nasal cavity
Upper respiratory tract
The upper respiratory tract warms and humidifies the air.
Nasopharynx
Oropharynx
Laryngopharynx
Pharynx
Epiglottis
Covers airway to prevent aspiration
Larynx
The larynx connects the upper and lower airways.
Left and right primary bronchi
Trachea
Carina
Cough reflex site
Lower respiratory tract
Alveoli
The alveoli are the primary gas exchange units of of the lungs.
Bronchioles
Alveolar duct
The lower airways terminate at the alveoli ducts.
Capillary
Alveolar sac
QUINN

What You Need to Know

Upper and Lower Respiratory Tract—Breathing Versus Gas Exchange

PULMONARY SYSTEM

The upper and lower airways, connected by the larynx, provide the passage of air into the lungs for gas exchange.

Upper Airway

- The nose and oropharynx are lined with ciliated mucosa that filters, humidifies, and warms the incoming air.
- Epiglottis and internal laryngeal muscles coordinate swallowing and inspiration to prevent aspiration.

Lower Airway

- Trachea, which conducts air into the lungs, connects the larynx to the bronchi.
- Trachea bifurcates at the carina to form the right and left bronchi. The right bronchus is straighter and shorter than the left bronchus. If a particle is aspirated, it will most likely go down the right bronchus.
- Carina is sensitive to foreign matter, protects against aspiration, and is the gag reflex site.
- Bronchioles terminate in the alveoli for gas exchange.

Gas Exchange

- Alveoli are the primary areas for gas exchange. Oxygen enters the blood and carbon dioxide is released from the blood across the alveolocapillary membrane.
- Pores of Kohn allow air to be distributed evenly across the alveoli.
- Surfactant is a defense mechanism that allows the alveoli to expand during inspiration and keeps the alveoli free of fluids.
- Pulmonary circulation receives blood through the pulmonary artery from the right ventricle. The vessels branch through the bronchi and eventually form arterioles at the alveolar level. The network of arteriole capillaries eventually end in the alveolocapillary membrane for gas exchange. A pulmonary embolus may lodge in the vessels of the pulmonary circulation.
- Bronchial circulation is made up of veins and arteries that do not participate in gas exchange. This part of the systemic circulation provides nutrients to the conducting airway.

Important nursing implications | Serious/life-threatening implications

Most frequent side effects | Patient teaching

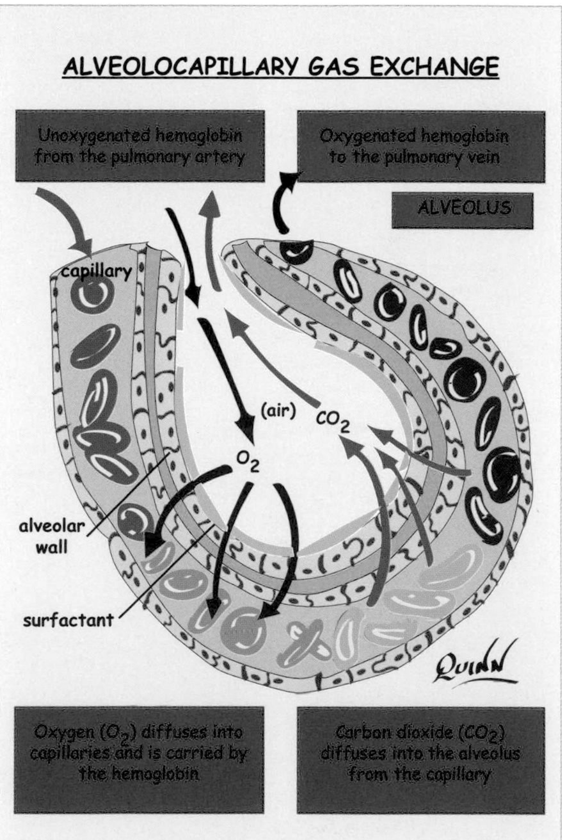
ALVEOLOCAPILLARY GAS EXCHANGE
Unoxygenated hemoglobin from the pulmonary artery
Oxygenated hemoglobin to the pulmonary vein
ALVEOLUS
capillary
(air)
CO_2
O_2
alveolar wall
surfactant
Quinn
Oxygen (O_2) diffuses into capillaries and is carried by the hemoglobin
Carbon dioxide (CO_2) diffuses into the alveolus from the capillary

What You Need to Know

Alveolocapillary Gas Exchange

SIGNIFICANCE OF ALVEOLOCAPILLARY GAS EXCHANGE

The lungs facilitate gas exchange between the circulatory system and the external environment.

CONTROL OF GAS EXCHANGE

Control of gas exchange takes place at the alveolar membrane. Oxygen and carbon dioxide are transported mainly by hemoglobin and exchanged through the capillary membrane by diffusion.

- Oxygen enters the capillary membrane and begins to dissolve in plasma. As it dissolves, pressure is exerted, which is known as the partial pressure of oxygen in arterial blood (PaO_2). As the PaO_2 increases, oxygen binds to red blood cells (RBCs) and attaches itself to hemoglobin molecules until the molecules become saturated.
- Oxygen saturation is expressed as a percentage—95% oxygen saturation means that 95% of the hemoglobin molecules have oxygen attached to them. Normal oxygen saturation is 92%–100%.
- Carbon dioxide is a product of cellular metabolism. It diffuses into the hemoglobin, is returned to the lungs where it moves across the alveolocapillary membrane into the alveoli, and is exhaled during respiration. At the cellular level, a drop in the oxygen saturation increases the ability of hemoglobin to carry carbon dioxide back to the alveoli.

ALVEOLOCAPILLARY MEMBRANE

- Allows the blood in the capillary to be exposed to the air or gas in the alveoli. Oxygen diffuses into the RBCs, and carbon dioxide diffuses out of the RBCs into the alveoli.
- The alveolar membrane is very fragile and easily damaged. Damage to this membrane allows blood and plasma to move into the alveolar spaces.
- Alveolar cells secrete surfactant that covers the inside of the alveoli, promotes the expansion of the alveoli during inspiration, and prevents collapse of the alveoli on expiration.
- Hypoxia is decreased tissue oxygenation.
- Hypoxemia is low levels of oxygen in the arterial blood.

COMMON MANIFESTATIONS OF PULMONARY DISEASE

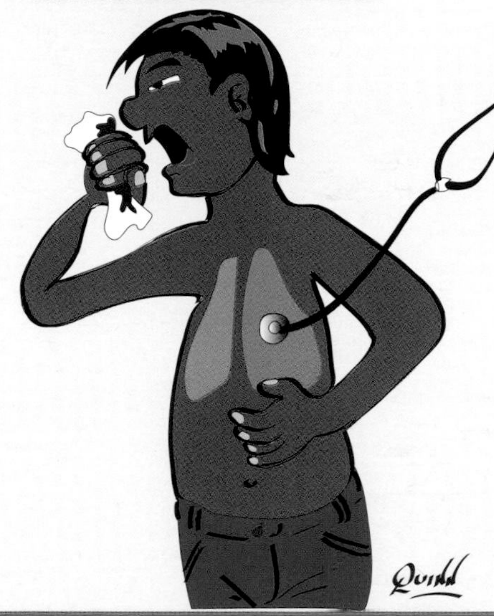

SYMPTOMS OF PULMONARY DISEASE

Lungs Sounds	Breathing Patterns	Physical Characteristics
Wheezing (whistle)	Dyspnea (short of breath)	Cough
Rhonchi (coarse)	Hypoventilation (pH < 7.4) Acidosis	Hemoptysis (bloody sputum)
Rales (crackles)	Hyperventilation (pH > 7.4) Alkalosis	Cyanosis
Diminished (soft)		Clubbing
		Pleural pain

What You Need to Know

Common Manifestations of Pulmonary Disease

SIGNIFICANCE OF PULMONARY DISEASE

Pulmonary disease is classified as acute or chronic, obstructive or restrictive, and infectious or noninfectious.

- Dyspnea (shortness of breath) and cough are common.
  - Feels as though the person cannot catch his or her breath.
  - Nostrils are flared.
  - Breathing is labored.
- Types of dyspnea
  - Dyspnea on exertion (DOE)—occurs with or during increased physical activity.
  - Paroxysmal nocturnal dyspnea (PND)—occurs with left ventricular failure. The patient will wake up in the middle of the night gasping for air.
  - Orthopnea—occurs while lying down and is usually relieved when sitting up.

ABNORMAL BREATHING PATTERNS AND LUNG SOUNDS

Abnormal Breathing Patterns

- *Eupnea* is normal breathing that is effortless and at a rate of 8–16 breaths per minute.
- *Tachypnea* is rapid breathing at a rate greater than 16 breaths per minute.
- *Bradypnea* is slow breathing at a rate of less than 8 breaths per minute.
- *Apnea* is cessation of breathing.

When the rate, depth, regularity, and effort of breathing change, abnormal breathing patterns occur.

Lung Sounds

- Wheeze—high-pitched squeaking sounds usually heard on expiration that are caused by bronchospasm and evident with asthma, airway obstruction, or COPD.
- Rhonchi—snoring sound that may be caused by cystic fibrosis, COPD, or bronchiectasis.
- Fine crackles—high-pitched sounds heard just before the end of inspiration caused by pulmonary edema, early stage of congestive heart failure (CHF), pneumonia, or atelectasis.

- Coarse crackles—short, low-pitched sounds heard on inspiration and expiration. The sound is similar to that of blowing through a straw under water. Coarse crackles are caused by air moving through fluid; they occur in pneumonia, COPD, CHF, and pulmonary edema.
- Stridor—continuous musical sound with a constant pitch that is caused by narrow airway. It occurs in croup, epiglottitis, or foreign-body aspiration.

Important nursing implications
Serious/life-threatening implications
Most frequent side effects
Patient teaching

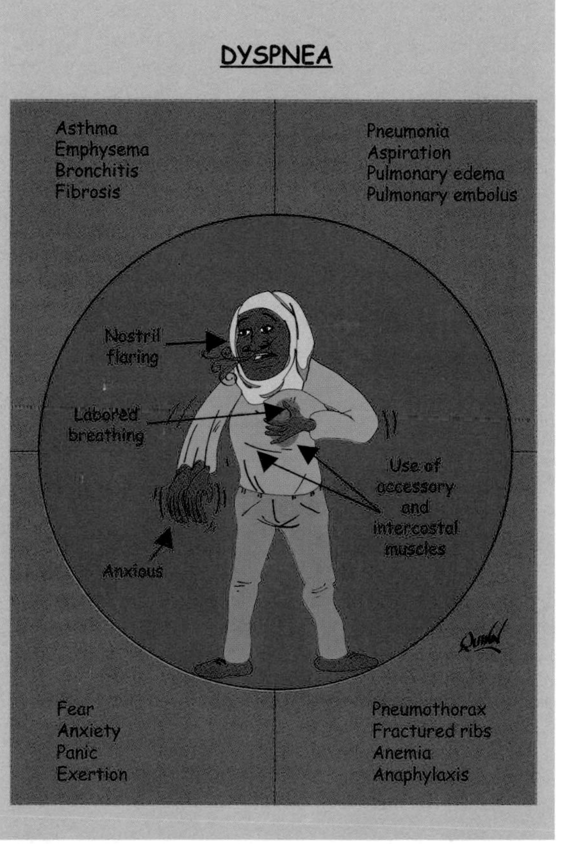
DYSPNEA
Asthma
Emphysema
Bronchitis
Fibrosis
Pneumonia
Aspiration
Pulmonary edema
Pulmonary embolus
Nostril flaring
Labored breathing
Use of accessory and intercostal muscles
Anxious
Fear
Anxiety
Panic
Exertion
Pneumothorax
Fractured ribs
Anemia
Anaphylaxis

What You Need to Know

Dyspnea

SIGNIFICANCE OF DYSPNEA

Dyspnea is a subjective breathing experience. The patient perceives having difficulty breathing; reports an "uncomfortable" feeling or not being able to "catch my breath."

CAUSES

- Increased airway resistance—most commonly seen in patients with COPD.
    - Asthma—airway is inflamed with increased vascular permeability and edema formation. Tenacious mucus makes breathing more labored and expiration more difficult.
    - Emphysema—alveoli become enlarged and lose their elasticity, which causes a trapping of air in the alveolar sacs.
    - Chronic bronchitis—inflammation, thickening, and swelling of mucus membranes occurs with increased amounts of mucus, which can lead to mucus plugs.
    - Anaphylaxis—hypersensitivity reaction, resulting in severe laryngeal edema, bronchospasm, and vascular collapse.
- Alveolar problems
    - Pneumonia—infection of the lung parenchyma causing alveoli to be inflamed
    - Aspiration—foreign substances in airways and lungs
    - Pneumothorax—complete or partial collapse of lung caused by air in the pleural space
    - Pulmonary edema—accumulation of fluid in the alveoli and interstitial spaces of the lungs

SIGNS AND SYMPTOMS

- Breathlessness, air hunger, shortness of breath
- Retraction of the accessory muscles in intercostal spaces
- Nostril flaring
- Cyanosis—bluish appearance of skin as a result of lack of oxygen in the blood (late sign)
- Labored breathing

    - Kussmaul respirations, as seen in patients with diabetic ketoacidosis (DKA)
    - Cheyne-Stokes respirations—alternating periods of deep breathing, shallow breathing, and periods of apnea
- PND—patient awakens at night with shortness of breath.
- Orthopnea—patient finds it easier to breathe sitting up.
- Hypoxemia—pulse oximetry may show a decreased level of oxygen saturation.

Important nursing implications | Serious/life-threatening implications
Most frequent side effects | Patient teaching

RESPIRATORY ACIDOSIS vs ALKALOSIS

RESPIRATORY ACIDOSIS SYMPTOMS

- Hypoventilation
- Hypercapnia
- Headache
- Drowsiness, dizziness, confusion
- Weakness
- Cardiac dysrhythmias
- Hypotension
- Hyperkalemia

RESPIRATORY ALKALOSIS SYMPTOMS

- Hyperventilation
- Hypocapnia
- Deep, rapid respirations
- Seizure
- Light headedness, lethargy, confusion
- Paresthesia of extremities
- Nausea, vomiting
- Hypotension or normotension
- Hypokalemia

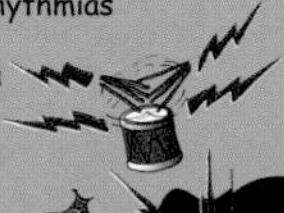

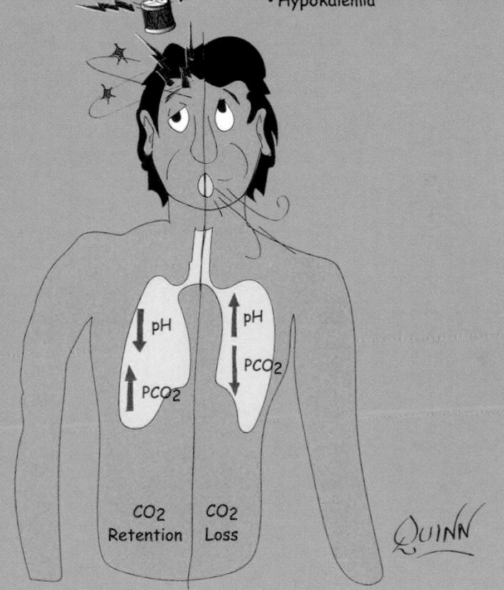

What You Need to Know

Respiratory Acidosis Versus Alkalosis

SIGNIFICANCE OF HYPERCAPNIA AND HYPOCAPNIA

In a state of hypoventilation, the body produces more carbon dioxide (CO_2) than it can eliminate, causing retention of CO_2. *Hypercapnia* is an increase in the partial pressure of arterial CO_2 ($PaCO_2$), often as a result of hypoventilation causing respiratory acidosis. *Hypocapnia* is a decreased $PaCO_2$ resulting from hyperventilation causing respiratory alkalosis.

CAUSES OF HYPERCAPNIA AND RESPIRATORY ACIDOSIS

- COPD; sleep apnea; ventilation-perfusion abnormalities; obesity; neuromuscular diseases
- Narcotic overdose or anesthesia

SIGNS AND SYMPTOMS OF RESPIRATORY ACIDOSIS

- pH less than 7.35; hypoventilation, hyperkalemia, and hypernatremia
- Change in mentation (confusion and lethargy); restlessness
- Cerebral vasodilation causing morning headache
- Hypotension; cardiac arrhythmias

CAUSES OF HYPOCAPNIA AND RESPIRATORY ALKALOSIS

- Anxiety or panic disorder; severe anemia; head injury or trauma
- High altitudes

SIGNS AND SYMPTOMS OF RESPIRATORY ALKALOSIS

- pH greater than 7.45; hyperventilation
- Hypokalemia
- Lightheadedness or lethargy; nausea; tremor; paresthesia

DIAGNOSTIC FINDINGS

- ABG—respiratory acidosis: ↓ pH; ↑ pCO_2 respiratory alkalosis ↑ pH; ↓ pCO_2

NURSING IMPLICATIONS

- Prevention—encourage the patient to turn, cough, and deep breathe.
- Maintain adequate hydration to increase removal of secretions.
- Use narcotics carefully, especially immediately postoperatively.
- Monitor for hyperkalemia.

HYPOXEMIA

Hypoventilation

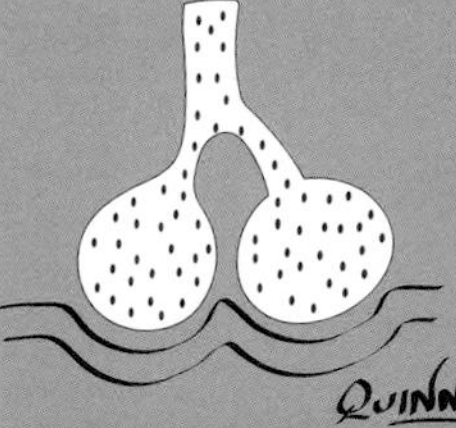

Hypoventilation

A decrease in respiratory drive.

Causes: Opioid intoxication, brain pathology (brain stem stroke), upper airway obstruction (epiglottis), neuromuscular weakness (Guillain Barre'), chronic respiratory mechanical problem (chronic obesity hypoxic syndrome).

V/Q mismatch

Partial obstruction of alveoli.

Causes: Asthma, COPD, pulmonary embolism, pulmonary edema, bronchopneumonia, most interstitial lung disease, heart failure.

V/Q mismatch

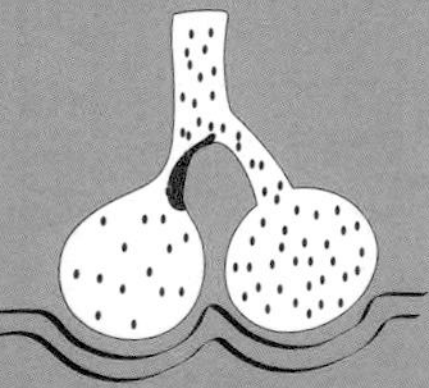

Shunt

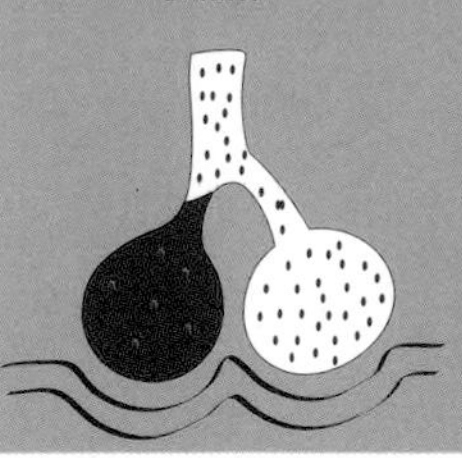

Shunt

Defective alveoli filling processes from lung consolidation.

Causes: Large bronchus obstruction from fluid (effusion), infection (pneumonia), atelectasis, ARDS, or vascular shunt.

What You Need to Know

Hypoxemia

SIGNIFICANCE OF HYPOXEMIA

Hypoxemia is a decrease in the oxygen saturation of the arterial blood (SaO_2). It results in a reduction of the oxygen available to tissue and body organs. This reduction occurs when the PaO_2 is decreased enough to cause signs and symptoms of poor oxygenation.

CAUSES

- *Decrease in inspired oxygen*—occurs in high altitudes or with suffocation.
- *Hypoventilation*—occurs in neurologic conditions during which the stimulus to breathe is impaired (oversedation, recovery from anesthetic, neurologic damage).
- *Impaired alveolocapillary diffusion*—when the alveolar membrane is compromised, an inadequate diffusion of oxygen occurs in the pulmonary capillary (i.e., thickening of the alveoli in emphysema, pulmonary fibrosis, and acute respiratory distress syndrome [ARDS]).
- *Shunting*—occurs when the blood returns from the lungs and is pumped from the heart without adequate oxygenation. This inadequacy occurs in an anatomic shunt (right-to-left shunt in congenital heart conditions) and in pulmonary edema, during which the alveoli are filled with fluid and in atelectasis.
- *Ventilation-perfusion mismatch (V/Q)*—occurs in conditions during which either the flow of oxygen is limited in the alveoli or the circulation through the pulmonary capillary is compromised (e.g., embolus).

SIGNS AND SYMPTOMS OF HYPOXIA SECONDARY TO HYPOXEMIA

- Dyspnea, tachypnea
- Headache
- Apprehension, confusion, lethargy
- Cyanosis of the nail beds and lips; discoloration of mucus membranes
- Dysrhythmias—tachycardia, premature ventricular contractions (PVCs), and premature atrial contractions (PACs)

DIAGNOSTIC FINDINGS

- PaO_2 level less than 80 mm Hg
- SaO_2 (arterial oxygen saturation) level less than 90%
- SpO_2 (pulse oximetry) level less than 92%

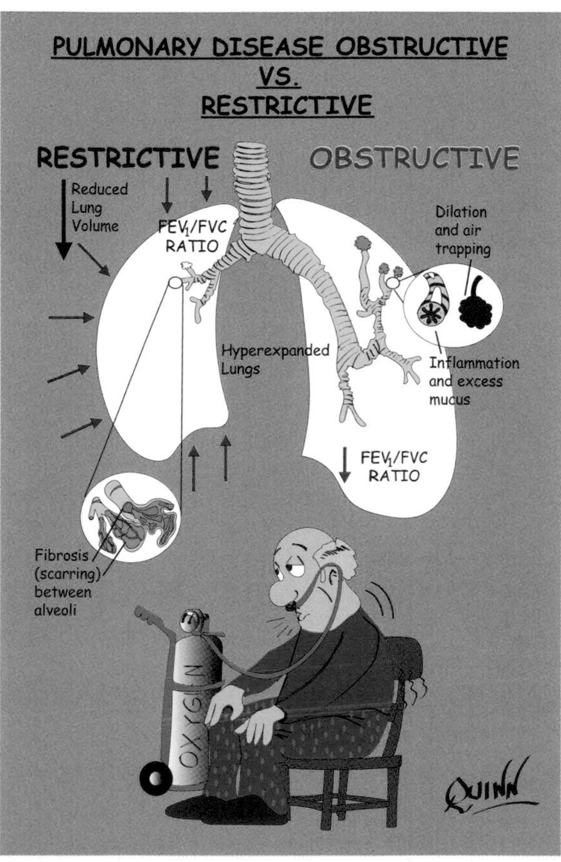
PULMONARY DISEASE OBSTRUCTIVE
VS.
RESTRICTIVE
RESTRICTIVE
OBSTRUCTIVE
Reduced
Lung
Volume
FEV1/FVC
RATIO
Dilation
and air
trapping
Hyperexpanded
Lungs
Inflammation
and excess
mucus
FEV1/FVC
RATIO
Fibrosis
(scarring)
between
alveoli
OXYGEN
QUINN

What You Need to Know

Pulmonary Disease: Obstructive Versus Restrictive Lung Disease

SIGNIFICANCE OF OBSTRUCTIVE AND RESTRICTIVE LUNG DISEASE

Chronic lung diseases (obstructive and restrictive) are characterized by an inflammatory condition involving the airways, lung parenchyma, and pulmonary vasculature. Both obstructive and restrictive lung disease lead to tissue destruction, airflow limitations, and impaired gas exchange. Obstructive lung disease is seen with the destruction of alveolar sacs and loss of elastic recoil. Whereas fibrotic thickening of the alveoli septae causing impaired gas is associated with restrictive lung disease. Obstructive and restrictive disease cause gradual increases in $PaCO_2$ and decreases in SaO_2.

CAUSES

- Obstructive: inhaled irritants, cigarette smoking, alpha-1 antitrypsin deficiency
- Restrictive: interstitial pulmonary fibrosis; sarcoidosis; cryptogenic organizing pneumonia

SIGNS AND SYMPTOMS

- Obstructive: Chronic and progressive dyspnea, cough, sputum production, orthopnea, wheezing, digital clubbing, cyanosis, pleuritic chest pain, hyperinflated lungs, barrel chest
- Restrictive: dyspnea, hypoxemia, bibasilar inspiratory crackles

DIAGNOSTIC FINDINGS

- ABG levels to identify acidosis or alkalosis
- Low serum potassium; possible positive alpha-1 antitrypsin; sputum culture to identify respiratory infections
- Pulmonary function test (PFT)
  - COPD: decreased ratio (<70%) of forced expiratory volume in 1 second to forced vital capacity (FEV1/FVC); total lung capacity (TLC) and FVC are usually normal
  - Restrictive: decreased TLC (<80%), FVC, and diffusing capacity for carbon dioxide (DLCO); preserved FEV1/FVC ratio (>70%)
- Six-minute walk test to determine need for oxygen
- High resolution CT for restrictive lung disease showing “honeycomb” pattern

NURSING MANAGEMENT

- Promote and teach good pulmonary hygiene including taking deep breaths.
- Administer the level of oxygen necessary to treat hypoxia and be ready to provide respiratory support.
- Monitor the patient for the development of right-sided heart failure.

Important nursing implications
Serious/life-threatening implications
Most frequent side effects
Patient teaching

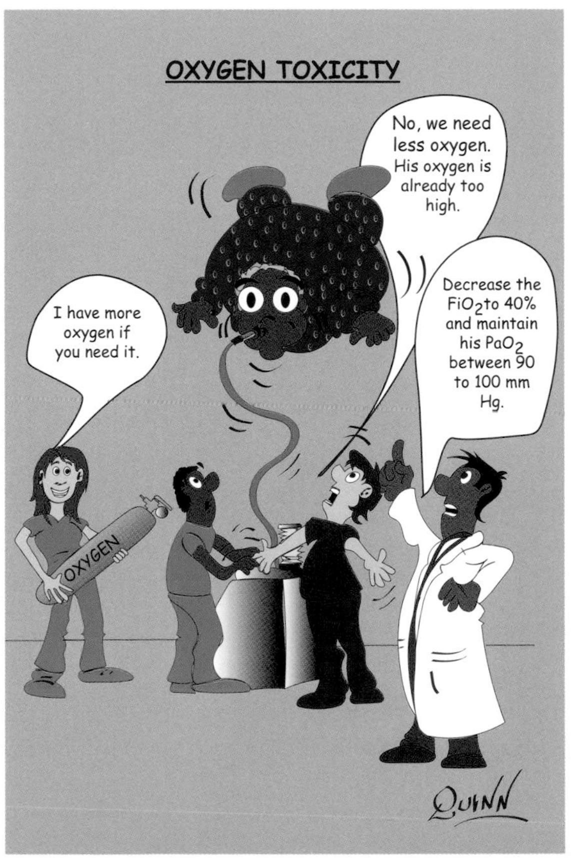
OXYGEN TOXICITY
I have more oxygen if you need it.
No, we need less oxygen. His oxygen is already too high.
Decrease the FiO_2 to 40% and maintain his PaO_2 between 90 to 100 mm Hg.
OXYGEN
QUINN

What You Need to Know

Oxygen Toxicity

SIGNIFICANCE OF OXYGEN TOXICITY

Oxygen toxicity can occur in any individual who requires extended exposure to above normal oxygen partial pressures, or shorter exposures to very high partial pressures. Normal oxygen ABG (SaO_2) is 92%–100%. Oxygen toxicity stimulates an inflammatory reaction and damage to the alveolocapillary membranes including pulmonary edema, congestion, injury, and intraalveolar hemorrhage.

CAUSES

- Most often seen in critical care settings:
  - Intubation and mechanical ventilation with high FiO_2
  - High-oxygen concentrations for an extended period (premature infants)
- Patients should receive the lowest level of oxygen necessary to keep the PaO_2 level within normal limits.

SIGNS AND SYMPTOMS

- Dry cough, dyspnea, pleural or substernal chest pain brought on by deep inhalation
- Nasal stuffiness, sore throat, malaise, fatigue
- Gastrointestinal (GI) upset
- Central nervous system oxygen toxicity causes visual changes, tinnitus, nausea, twitching, and behavioral changes

Toxicity may be undetected, secondary to the patient's respiratory condition. The clinical manifestations of oxygen toxicity are often difficult to differentiate from ARDS.

NURSING IMPLICATIONS

- Prevention is important. Closely monitor patients receiving oxygen and notify the healthcare provider for consistently high PaO_2 levels.
- Do not withhold high percentages of oxygen if patient is severely hypoxic. Oxygen toxicity is not as great a threat to life as hypoxemia.

Important nursing implications | Serious/life-threatening implications
Most frequent side effects | Patient teaching

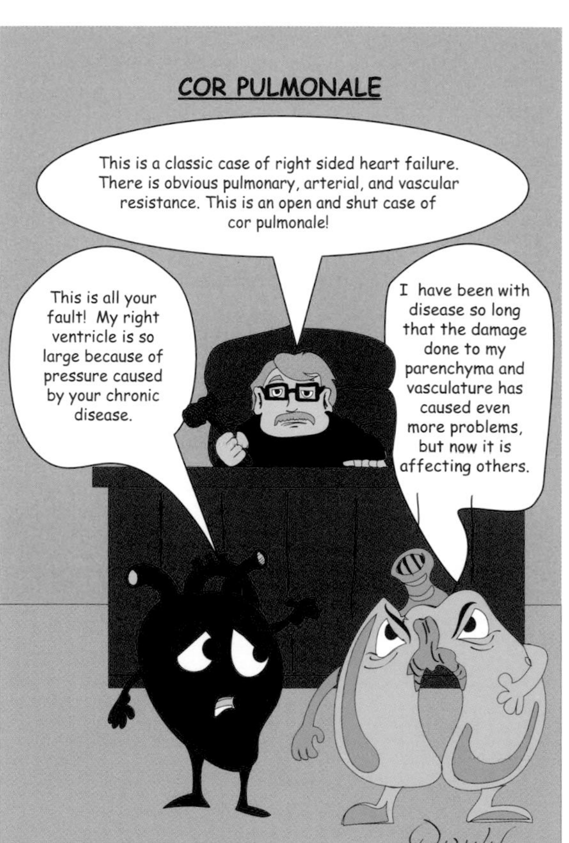
COR PULMONALE
This is a classic case of right sided heart failure. There is obvious pulmonary, arterial, and vascular resistance. This is an open and shut case of cor pulmonale!
This is all your fault! My right ventricle is so large because of pressure caused by your chronic disease.
I have been with disease so long that the damage done to my parenchyma and vasculature has caused even more problems, but now it is affecting others.
QUINN

What You Need to Know

Cor Pulmonale (Right-Sided Heart Failure)

SIGNIFICANCE OF COR PULMONALE

Right-sided heart failure most frequently occurs secondary to left-sided heart failure. When right-sided heart failure occurs alone, it is the result of increased pressure in the lung tissue, which places an increased workload on the heart to pump blood through the pulmonary vessels. It is commonly referred to as *cor pulmonale*. With an increased workload on the right ventricle, the ventricle enlarges, thickens, and begins to fail. The symptoms are predominantly systemic because of an increase in the venous pressure.

CAUSES

- Chronic obstructive pulmonary disease (emphysema, chronic bronchitis)
- Pulmonary embolus
- Chronic pulmonary arterial hypertension
- Pulmonary interstitial or cystic fibrosis
- Systemic sclerosis (scleroderma)
- Kyphoscoliosis

SIGNS AND SYMPTOMS

- Pulmonary symptoms
  - Increasing dyspnea
  - Wheezing and coughing
  - Hypoxia
- Cardiac symptoms
  - Peripheral edema
  - Jugular vein distention; bounding pulse; loud S2; murmur of tricuspid; S4 right-sided
  - Cyanotic hands and feet
  - Hepatomegaly; ascites

DIAGNOSTIC FINDINGS

- Presence of chronic pulmonary disease
- Evaluate for abnormal chest X-ray, electrocardiogram, echocardiography, or pulmonary function tests

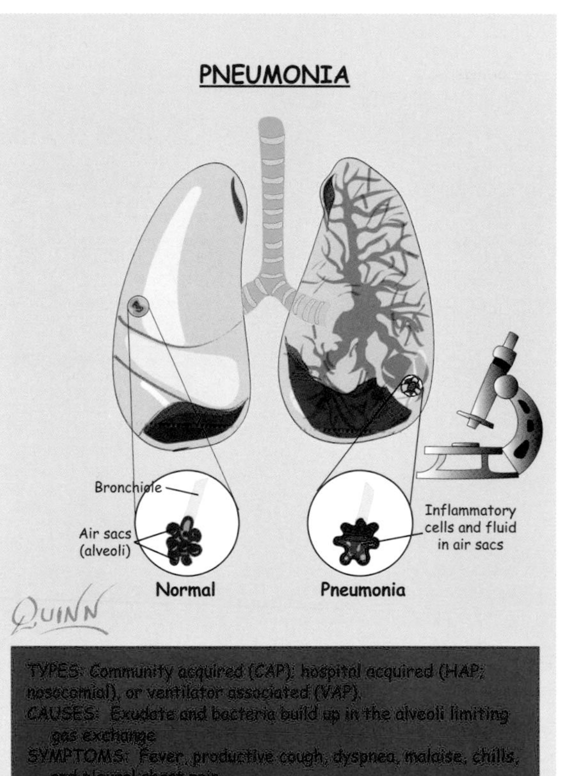
PNEUMONIA
Bronchiole
Air sacs
(alveoli)
Inflammatory
cells and fluid
in air sacs
Normal
Pneumonia
QUINN
TYPES: Community acquired (CAP); hospital acquired (HAP; nosocomial), or ventilator associated (VAP).
CAUSES: Exudate and bacteria build up in the alveoli limiting gas exchange
SYMPTOMS: Fever, productive cough, dyspnea, malaise, chills, and pleural chest pain
PREVENTION: Pneumonia vaccine, cover mouth when coughing, and handwashing.

What You Need to Know

Pneumonia

SIGNIFICANCE OF PNEUMONIA

Pneumonia occurs when a bacterial or viral pathogen invades the lung parenchyma at the alveolar level. The inflammatory response causes fluid, edema, and exudate to collect in the alveoli, causing a decrease in oxygenation and tissue perfusion.

CAUSES

- Community-acquired pneumonia (CAP) is acquired from the community or within 48 hours of hospital admission.
  - *Streptococcus pneumoniae* is the most common bacteria associated with CAP.
- Hospital-acquired pneumonia (HAP; nosocomial) develops after 48 hours of hospitalization. HAP also includes pneumonia acquired from healthcare facilities (e.g., nursing homes).
  - Methicillin-resistant *Staphylococcus aureus* (MRSA) and *Pseudomonas aeruginosa* are the most common pathogens associated with HAP.
- Ventilator-associated pneumonia (VAP) develops 48 hours or longer after intubation for mechanical ventilation.
  - *S. pneumoniae* and *Haemophilus influenzae* (multidrug resistant pathogens) are the most common pathogens associated with VAP.
- Viral pneumonia
  - *Respiratory syncytial virus (RSV); Rhinovirus,* and Human *Coronavirus* are most common viruses associated with viral pneumonia.

SIGNS AND SYMPTOMS

- Productive cough—mucoid, purulent, or blood-tinged
- Fever—lower in viral infection, chills, sweats, fatigue, pleuritic chest pain, headache, myalgia
- Dyspnea, tachypnea, orthopnea, breath sounds with crackles and wheezing
- Chest pain, tachycardia
- Rash—more common for viral pneumonia and in children

DIAGNOSTIC FINDINGS

- Chest X-ray, CBC, inflammatory markers, rapid antigen tests (RSV, influenza, coronavirus)

NURSING IMPLICATIONS—PREVENTION

- Hand hygiene is the most important action to prevent pneumonia.
- Provide patient education on the importance of vaccines, hand hygiene, covering mouth when coughing, and respiratory hygiene, especially for immobilized patients.
- Identify patients in hospital with high-risk factors, prevent cross-contamination of equipment, and verify the placement of endotracheal and nasogastric tubes.

Important nursing implications | Serious/life-threatening implications

Most frequent side effects | Patient teaching

COMMON SYMPTOMS OF CARDIAC PROBLEMS

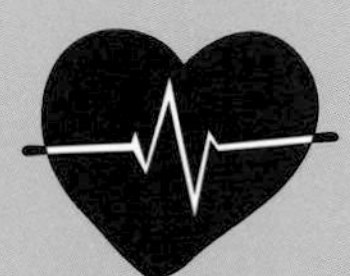

Normal heart rate: The normal heart rate (pulse) in adults is 60–80 beats per minute. The pulse rate can increase with exercise, illness, injury, and emotions.

Bradycardia: <60 beats per minute
Causes: Heart block, medication, electrolytes, hypoxia, stroke

Tachycardia: >100 beats per minute
Causes: Exercise, anemia, dehydration, fever, infection, drugs

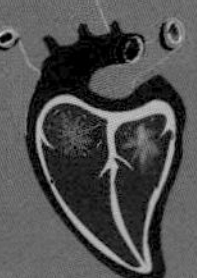

Dysrhythmia: A disturbance in the heart rhythm caused by disorganized electrical signals sent by the sinoatrial node or cells in the myocardium.

Ischemia: Interruption of arterial blood flow leads to tissue hypoxia, ischemic pain, alteration in the level of consciousness and decreased blood pressure and pulse rate.

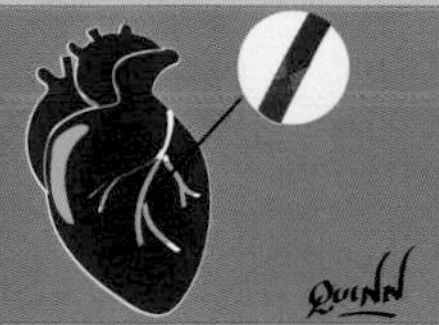

What You Need to Know

Common Symptoms of Cardiac Problems

SIGNIFICANCE OF HEART RATE

The normal heart rate (HR) is 60–100 beats per minute (bpm) with an average of 60–80 bpm. An increased HR increases the oxygen consumption of the myocardium. The parasympathetic nervous system slows the HR, and the sympathetic nervous system speeds up the HR.

FACTORS AFFECTING HEART RATE

- Neural reflexes cause the HR to increase or decrease with an infusion of blood or intravenous (IV) fluids. If the initial HR is slow, IV infusions will increase the HR. If the HR is rapid, then IV infusions will decrease the HR.
- Cardiovascular control center in medulla—synapses with the parasympathetic and sympathetic nervous systems.
- Baroreceptor reflexes—receive messages from the pressure receptors in the aortic arch and carotid sinus.
    - if blood pressure (BP) is down, vasoconstriction occurs and the HR increases.
    - if BP is elevated, vasodilation occurs, causing reduced contractility and subsequent reduced cardiac output (CO).
- Atrial receptors—are located in both atria. Distention of these receptors influences the HR—either increasing or decreasing it, based on the stimulus.
- Catecholamines (epinephrine and norepinephrine) will increase the HR.
- Excessive level of thyroid hormone causes tachycardia and hypertension.
- Resting HR is primarily under the control of the parasympathetic system.
- Obesity—increases the workload on the heart, which increases the HR.

DYSRHYTHMIAS

Dysrhythmias are a disturbance in the heart rhythm from the sinoatrial (SA) node or cells in the myocardium. Dysrhythmias can be either benign (missed beat) or serious (disturbance in the pumping ability, leading to heart failure).

- Ventricular fibrillation—significant decrease in CO occurs, and advanced cardiac life support must be initiated.
- Premature ventricular contractions (PVCs)—are early beats in the cardiac cycle. They are commonly caused by electrolyte imbalances (e.g., hyperkalemia), cardiac ischemia, and hypoxia.
- Bradycardia—pulse rate is lower than 60 bpm.
- Tachycardia—pulse rate is higher than 100 bpm.

CARDIAC OUTPUT

Heart Rate is measured in beats per minute.

Stroke Volume is the volume of blood ejected during systole.

Cardiac Output is determined by multiplying the heart rate by the stroke volume. Normal is about 5 L/min.

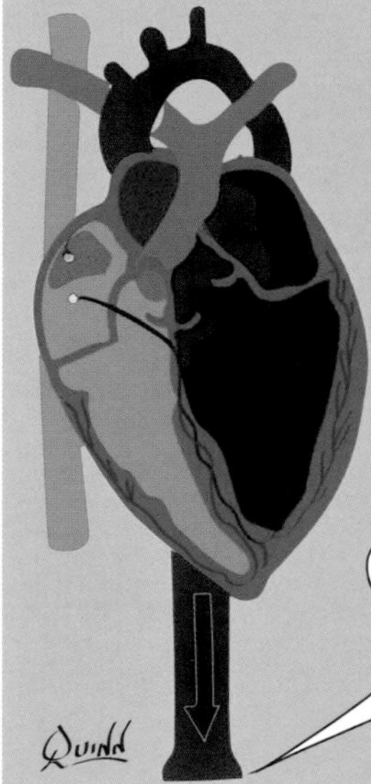

Cardiac output is the amount of blood ejected by the heart in 1 minute and is measured in liters.

Ventricular volume is measured by the filling pressure and ventricular compliance.

Filling pressure of the right ventricle is based on the right atrial pressure. Filling of the left ventricle is based on the left atrial pressure.

What You Need to Know

Cardiac Output

CO is the amount of blood ejected by the heart in 1 minute and is measured in liters. The CO is dependent on two factors: (1) HR and (2) stroke volume (SV) and is controlled by both. The SV is the measurement of the amount of blood ejected per minute during systole.

CALCULATING CARDIAC OUTPUT

$$CO = SV \times HR$$

- Decreased HR and increased SV cause an increase in CO.
- Increased HR and increased SV cause an increase in CO.
- Normal CO for an adult is 4–7 L/min.

CONTROL OF CARDIAC OUTPUT

- Factors affecting the SV:
  - *Preload*—is the amount of blood returning to the heart from the pulmonary vessels (left side) and the venous return (right side). The filling pressures of the ventricles are represented by the pressures in the right and left atria.
  - *Afterload*—is the resistance that the heart must overcome to pump blood through the valves and aorta to the peripheral circulation. Afterload is affected by the systemic vascular resistance (SVR), aortic compliance, and blood viscosity.
  - *Contractility*—is the amount of force generated by the myocardium to eject blood into circulation. Ventricular compliance and filling pressure affect the SV.
- Increasing CO:
  - Increased preload—blood returns to the right atrium.
  - Increased contractility occurs.
  - Decreased afterload—decreases pressure that the heart must pump against.
- Factors affecting the HR:
  - HR affects the CO by causing a decrease or increase in SV.
  - HR is controlled by baroreceptors in the aortic arch, which are sensitive to changes in the BP.
  - Stimulation of the parasympathetic nervous system (vagus nerve) decreases the HR.
  - Stimulation of the sympathetic nervous system increases the HR.

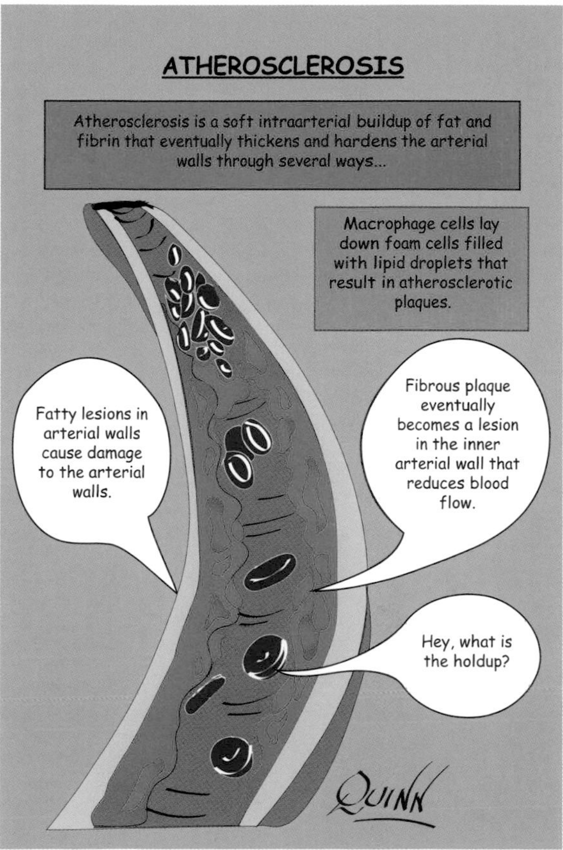
ATHEROSCLEROSIS
Atherosclerosis is a soft intraarterial buildup of fat and fibrin that eventually thickens and hardens the arterial walls through several ways...
Macrophage cells lay down foam cells filled with lipid droplets that result in atherosclerotic plaques.
Fatty lesions in arterial walls cause damage to the arterial walls.
Fibrous plaque eventually becomes a lesion in the inner arterial wall that reduces blood flow.
Hey, what is the holdup?
QUINN

What You Need to Know

Atherosclerosis

SIGNIFICANCE OF ATHEROSCLEROSIS

Atherosclerosis is not a single disease or problem. It is a process that affects the entire arterial vascular system and is the leading cause of coronary artery and cerebrovascular disease. Atherosclerosis is a hardening and thickening of the arterial walls caused by a buildup of plaque within the lining of the artery.

- Endothelial cells in the artery are injured and become inflamed.
- Ability to oxidize low-density lipoprotein (LDL) is impaired.
- Macrophages filled with oxidized LDL (foam cells) begin to adhere to the endothelium and produce fatty streaks that develop into plaques.
- Antithrombotic and vasodilating cytokines are not effective and the ability of the artery to remove the plaque becomes ineffective.
- Collagen forms over the fatty streak, and a fibrous plaque is formed.
- Fibrous plaque begins to impede blood flow, which causes inadequate tissue perfusion to vital organs.
- Plaques that rupture precipitate the adhesion of platelets and the development of a thrombus, which may suddenly occlude an artery, resulting in tissue ischemia and possible infarction and necrosis.

CAUSES OF ATHEROSCLEROSIS

- Consumption of high fat and cholesterol (LDL)-containing foods causing high cholesterol and triglyceride levels.
- Hypertension
- Diabetes mellitus, insulin resistance
- Smoking and obesity (inhibits the oxidation of LDL)
- Increased C-reactive protein, infection, and periodontal disease (these risk factors have been identified as possible causes of endothelial injury).

NURSING IMPLICATIONS

- Encourage the intake of enriched fortified cereals that contain folic acid, vitamin B6 (pyridoxine), and vitamin B12 (cyanocobalamine); encourage an increased intake of fresh vegetables. Discourage meals high in LDL (e.g., red meat, eggs, food fried in saturated fats).
- Teach the importance of regular exercise and weight management.
- Encourage patients with diabetes mellitus to maintain good glucose control.

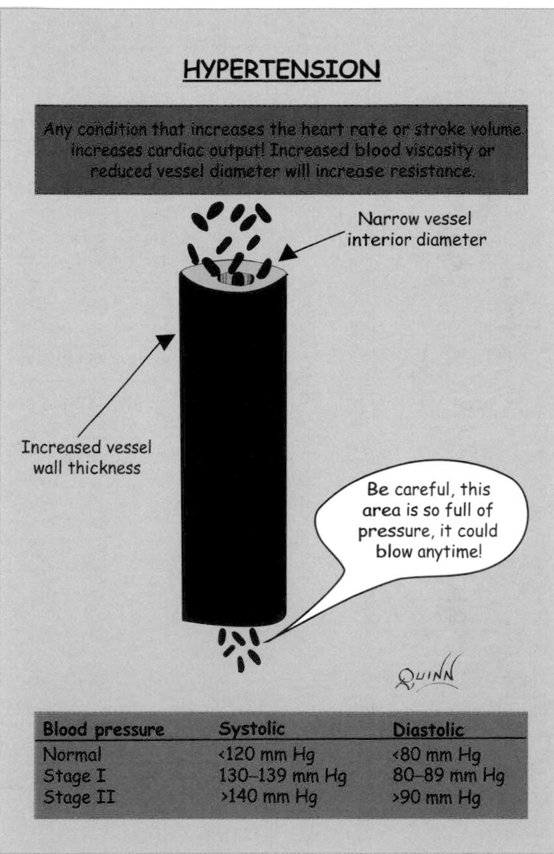

Blood pressure	Systolic	Diastolic
Normal	<120 mm Hg	<80 mm Hg
Stage I	130–139 mm Hg	80–89 mm Hg
Stage II	>140 mm Hg	>90 mm Hg

What You Need to Know

Hypertension

SIGNIFICANCE OF HYPERTENSION

Hypertension is the sustained elevation of BP. Hypertension is either primary or secondary. Normal BP is systolic <120 mm Hg and diastolic <80 mm Hg.

TYPES OF HYPERTENSION

Primary Hypertension

Elevated BP without a known causative factor is classified as primary hypertension. For an elevated BP to occur, the CO or SVR increases. Increased SVR is the hallmark sign of primary hypertension.

Causes of Primary Hypertension

- Genetic predisposition, obesity
- Stress, increased alcohol intake
- Diabetes mellitus, sodium and water retention

Secondary Hypertension

Elevated BP with an identifiable cause is classified as secondary hypertension. Patients who suddenly develop hypertension should have a complete history and physical examination. Further diagnostic evaluation may be necessary to evaluate for a secondary cause.

Causes of Secondary Hypertension

- Renal stenosis, chronic kidney disease
- Congenital heart defects (e.g., aortic coarctation)
- Cushing syndrome, pheochromocytoma, adrenal disease
- Untreated sleep apnea
- Monoamine oxidase inhibitors (MAOIs)
- Stimulants (e.g., cocaine, methamphetamines)
- Pregnancy-induced hypertension (preeclampsia)

SIGNS AND SYMPTOMS

Hypertension is often called the *silent killer* because initial symptoms are not frequently presented. Signs and symptoms include:

- Chronic fatigue
- Headache
- Dizziness
- Dyspnea at rest or with physical exertion
- Chest pain and palpitations

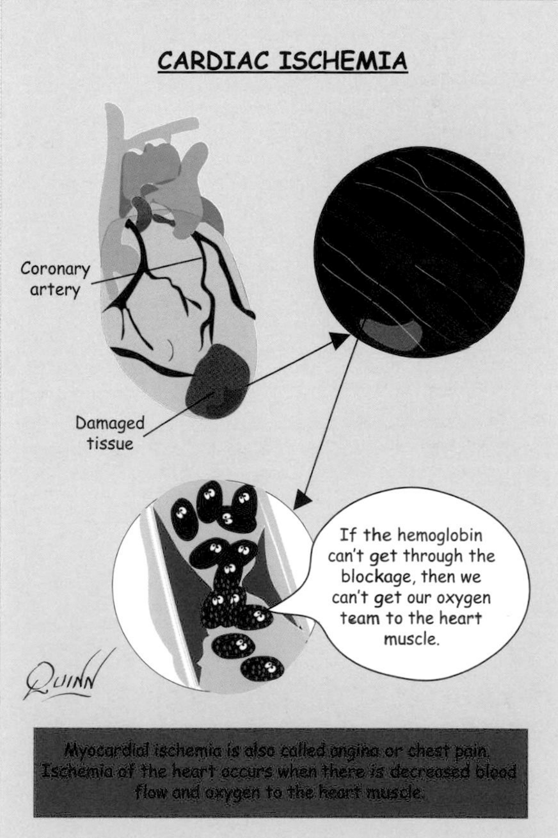
CARDIAC ISCHEMIA
Coronary artery
Damaged tissue
If the hemoglobin can't get through the blockage, then we can't get our oxygen team to the heart muscle.
QUINN
Myocardial ischemia is also called angina or chest pain. Ischemia of the heart occurs when there is decreased blood flow and oxygen to the heart muscle.

What You Need to Know

Cardiac Ischemia

SIGNIFICANCE OF ISCHEMIA

Ischemia is a decrease in blood supply and tissue oxygenation. Angina is chest pain caused by ischemia of the myocardium.

Atherosclerosis is the major cause of ischemia, resulting from a buildup of plaque, which causes occlusion.

- Occluded vessels decrease or obstruct blood flow to the heart.
- Pain occurs as a result of the buildup of lactic acid in the myocardium.
- In a severe ischemic environment, cardiac cells remain viable for approximately 20 minutes.
- Myocardial ischemia may be asymptomatic and "silent" with no chest pain.

TYPES OF CARDIAC ISCHEMIA

- Chronic stable angina most often occurs with an increase in exercise or activity.
  - Pain is caused by a gradual narrowing of an artery; consequently, the artery cannot respond to increased myocardial demand.
  - Pain may radiate to the lower neck, left shoulder, and arms; it may also be described as epigastric distress (heartburn).
  - Cessation of activity frequently relieves pain. The discomfort is transient and usually lasts for 3–5 minutes.
- Unstable angina occurs with severe cardiac ischemia. It may be reversible, but it may be indicative of impending myocardial infarction (MI).
  - Pain is present at rest.
  - Pain usually lasts longer than 15–20 minutes and is unrelieved by nitroglycerin.
  - Most often occurs as new-onset angina or angina that occurs at rest or increasingly severe angina.
- Prinzmetal angina—results from transient ischemia, is unpredictable, and frequently occurs at rest. It may be the result of arterial spasm.

DIAGNOSTIC FINDINGS

- ST segment depression and T-wave inversion are observed on the ECG strip.
- Exercise stress test results are positive.

- Single photon-emission computerized tomography (SPECT) results are positive.
- Coronary angiography shows vessel occlusion.
- After severe ischemia, cellular death occurs, which releases intracellular enzymes that can be measured.
    - Increased cardiac enzymes: troponin, CK, CK-MB

Important nursing implications | Serious/life-threatening implications
Most frequent side effects | Patient teaching

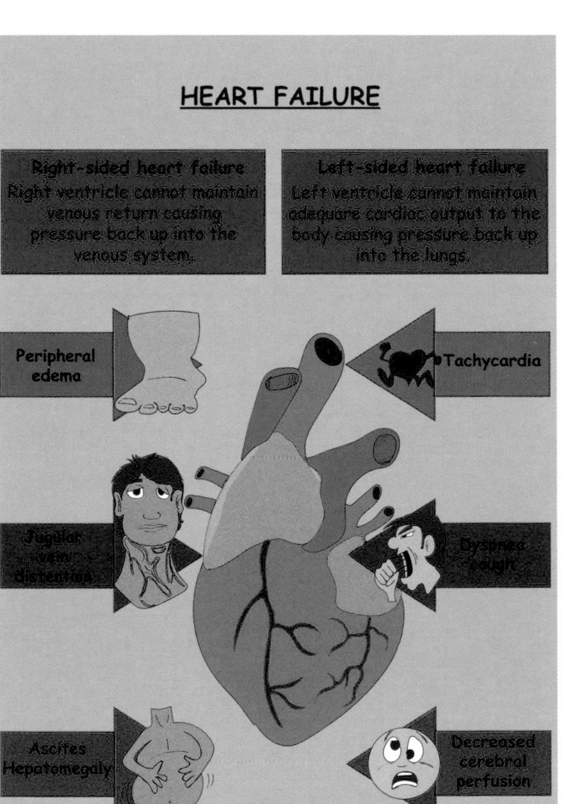
HEART FAILURE
Right-sided heart failure
Right ventricle cannot maintain venous return causing pressure back up into the venous system.
Left-sided heart failure
Left ventricle cannot maintain adequare cardiac output to the body causing pressure back up into the lungs.
Peripheral edema
Tachycardia
Jugular vein distention
Dyspnea cough
Ascites Hepatomegaly
Decreased cerebral perfusion
QUINN

What You Need to Know

Heart Failure

SIGNIFICANCE OF HEART FAILURE

Heart failure is the result of the inability of the heart to pump adequate amounts of blood into the systemic circulation to meet the metabolic demands of the tissues.

TYPES OF HEART FAILURE

Left-Sided (With Reduced Ejection Fraction [HFrEF] or With Preserved Ejection Fraction [HFpEF])

- Left side of the heart is unable to handle the blood return from the pulmonary vein.
- Pressure backs up into the pulmonary system.
- Left ventricle cannot maintain adequate CO in the body.
- Precipitating factors include MI, hypertension, aortic and mitral valve disease, and dysrhythmia.

Right-Sided

- Right side of the heart is unable to handle the blood return from systemic circulation.
- Pressure backs up into venous system.
- Right ventricle cannot maintain CO in the pulmonary system.
- Precipitating factors include left-sided heart failure and chronic pulmonary hypertension.

SIGNS AND SYMPTOMS

- Left-sided heart failure (signs of decreased organ perfusion)
  - Pulmonary congestion and edema (crackles, wheezing, tachypnea, frothy sputum)
  - Tachycardia
  - Decreased cerebral perfusion
  - Excessive fatigue
  - Dyspnea, orthopnea, cough
  - Nocturia; decreased urine output less than 30 mL/h
- Right-sided heart failure
  - Weight gain, jugular vein distention (JVD), tachycardia
  - Hepatomegaly, pain in upper right quadrant
  - Peripheral edema, ascites
  - Clear lungs, paradoxical pulse (BP increases on expiration)

VALVULAR DYSFUNCTION

Causes of Valve Disease

- Congenital heart disease
- Rheumatic fever
- Aging heart valves
- Infection (endocarditis)
- Trauma
- Ischemia

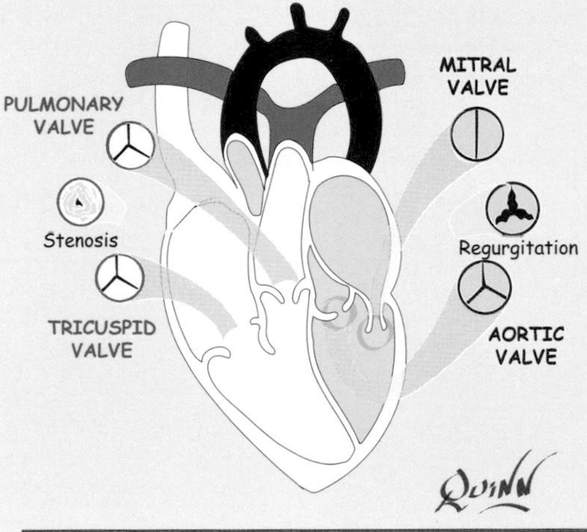

PULMONARY VALVE

Stenosis

TRICUSPID VALVE

MITRAL VALVE

Regurgitation

AORTIC VALVE

Quinn

REGURGITATION is the leaking or back flow of blood through the valve from a lack of closure.

STENOSIS is a smaller opening for blood to flow through the valve, which creates higher pressures.

What You Need to Know

Valvular Dysfunction

SIGNIFICANCE OF VALVULAR DYSFUNCTION

The four valves of the heart are the mitral, aortic, tricuspid, and pulmonary. The mitral and atrial valves are most affected for stenosis and regurgitation. When the heart cannot compensate for the valvular defects, heart failure develops.

VALVULAR STENOSIS

Stenosis refers to the constriction or narrowing of the valve's opening.

- Mitral valve stenosis
  - Mitral valve is constricted, causing increased pressure in the right atrium with increasing pulmonary artery pressure.
  - **Signs and symptoms**: Diastolic murmur, hemoptysis, and fatigue.
- Aortic valve stenosis
  - Aortic valve becomes narrowed, preventing normal blood flow from the left ventricle into the aorta during systole; decreases filling of the coronary arteries.
  - **Signs and symptoms**: Chest pain, crescendo-decrescendo murmur, dyspnea on exertion, syncope, and heart failure.

VALVULAR REGURGITATION

Regurgitation refers to the inability of the valve leaflets to close completely, causing the backward flow of blood.

- Mitral valve regurgitation.
  - Blood backs up (regurgitates) into the left atrium and causes hypertrophy and dilation of the left ventricle because of volume overload.
  - May be asymptomatic until left ventricular failure develops secondary to chronic volume overload.
  - **Signs and symptoms**: Weakness, dyspnea on exertion, orthopnea, and systolic murmur.
- Aortic valve regurgitation
  - Blood flows back into the left ventricle from the descending aorta, causing left ventricular overload and left ventricular hypertrophy.
  - **Signs and symptoms**: May be asymptomatic until left ventricular failure develops.

NURSING MANAGEMENT

- Teach the importance of preventing carditis and valvular damage by adequately treating rheumatic fever (RF) with antibiotics, and cessation of drugs (e.g., cocaine, heroin).
- If carditis occurs with RF, then the patient will need to continue taking prophylactic antibiotics, especially before invasive treatments.
- Teach the early signs of heart failure and the importance of maintaining regular checkups.
- Pregnant women with valve problems will begin to exhibit symptoms of heart failure, most often in the third trimester.

Important nursing implications   Serious/life-threatening implications

Most frequent side effects   Patient teaching

CARDIAC CONDUCTION SYSTEM

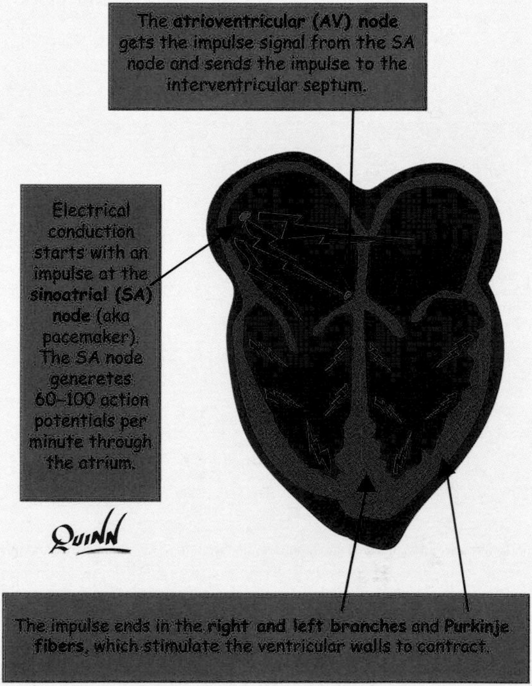

The **atrioventricular (AV) node** gets the impulse signal from the SA node and sends the impulse to the interventricular septum.

Electrical conduction starts with an impulse at the **sinoatrial (SA) node** (aka pacemaker). The SA node generetes 60–100 action potentials per minute through the atrium.

QUINN

The impulse ends in the **right and left branches** and **Purkinje fibers**, which stimulate the ventricular walls to contract.

What You Need to Know

Cardiac Conduction System

SIGNIFICANCE OF CARDIAC CONDUCTION SYSTEM

The SA node is the starting point for impulse formation. When the impulses are formed, they travel through the myocardium, initiating the contraction of the atria.

The impulses travel from the atria to the ventricular myocardium. These impulses travel through the atrioventricular (AV) node to the bundle of His and continue through the right and left bundle branches of the interventricular septum to the Purkinje fibers in the heart wall.

CARDIAC TISSUE PROPERTIES

Specialized cardiac cells have electrophysiologic properties that allow the cells to control the rate and rhythm of the heart.

- Automaticity—ability to initiate an impulse spontaneously and continuously
- Excitability—ability to be stimulated electrically
- Contractility—ability to respond mechanically to an impulse
- Conductivity—ability to transmit an impulse along a membrane

LOCATION OF CONDUCTION NODES

- SA node is located at the junction of the right atrium and the superior vena cava. The P wave is initiated by the SA node and should proceed every ventricular conduction (QRS) interval.
- AV junction—is located in the lower atrium above the tricuspid valve. AV node slows impulses to allow adequate ventricular filling after atrial conduction, which is reflected in the PR interval.
- Bundle of His extends down the right and left interventricular septa.
- Bundle branches conduct the impulse through the Purkinje fibers and initiate ventricular contraction.
- Purkinje fibers are located at the ends of the right and left bundle branches and extend out to the myocardium to initiate the contraction, which is reflected in the QRS interval.

Important nursing implications | Serious/life-threatening implications
Most frequent side effects | Patient teaching

PERIPHERAL ARTERIAL DISEASE

Peripheral arterial disease (PAD) is the narrowing of arteries in the extremities caused by plaque buildup and claudication. PAD increases risks of limb ischemia, myocardial ischemia, and stroke

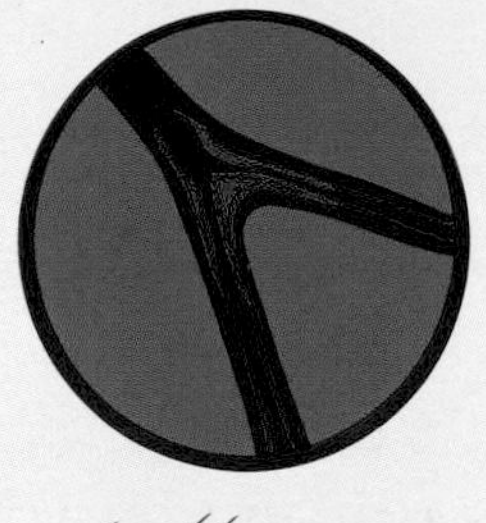

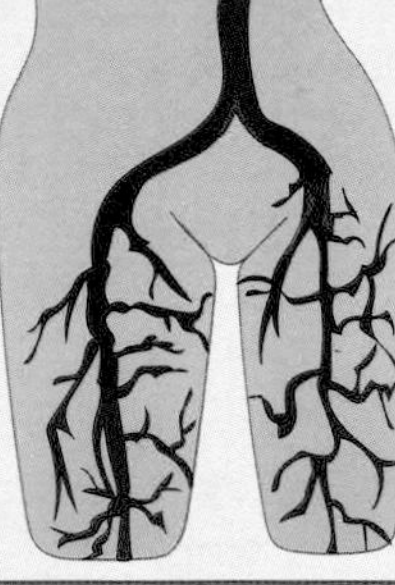

QUINN

Risk Factors:

- Atherosclerosis
- Hypertension
- Smoking
- Obesity
- Hyperlipidemia
- Diabetes
- Genetics
- Age

Symptoms:

- Pain
- Muscle fatigue
- Ulcers
- Unilateral discoloration
- Paresthesia
- Muscle cramping
- Open wounds
- Unilateral cool extremity

What You Need to Know

Peripheral Arterial Disease

SIGNIFICANCE OF PERIPHERAL ARTERIAL DISEASE

Peripheral arterial disease is commonly observed in the patient who has diabetes mellitus or is hypertensive or both. It most often occurs as a result of occlusion of arterial blood flow to the lower limbs by atherosclerosis, a gradual thickening of the intima and media of vessel walls. Peripheral artery disease increases the risk of limb ischemia, myocardial ischemia, and stroke.

SIGNS AND SYMPTOMS

- Most common in the lower extremities
- Weakened or absent pedal pulses
- Thick toenails
- Cool, pale, shiny skin with scaling present
- Absence of hair on lower extremities
- Poor wound healing; ulcerations over bony prominences
- Intermittent claudication (pain in lower extremities with exercise) relieved by rest

DIAGNOSTIC FINDINGS

- Angiography of extremity
- Doppler ultrasound
- Ankle-brachial index (ABI)

MEDICAL MANAGEMENT

- Antiplatelet agents (e.g., aspirin, Plavix)
- Decrease risk factors of atherosclerosis
- Slow progressive physical activity; walking is recommended
- Peripheral arterial bypass surgery

NURSING MANAGEMENT

- Encourage client to maintain proper foot care.
  - Wear closed-toed shoes.
  - Wash feet daily and pat dry (especially between the toes).
  - Keep toenails trimmed (avoid developing ingrown nails).
- Report any lesions or ulcers that do not heal.
- Do not apply heat, cold, or chemicals to lesions or ulcers on the feet.
- Do not wear constrictive clothing.

CONGENITAL HEART DEFECTS

Congenital heart defects are the most common type of birth defect. The structural problems arise from abnormal formation of the heart or major blood vessels.

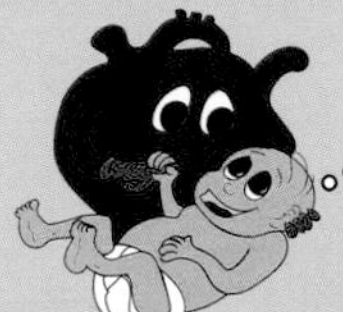

Lesions Increasing Pulmonary Blood Flow
(Acyanotic: Left-to-right shunt)

An unclosed hole in the aorta causes oxygenated blood to be shunted from the left side to the right side of the heart.

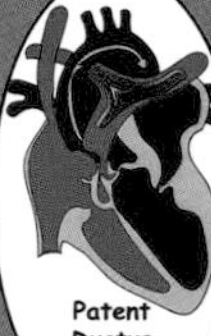

Lesions Decreasing Pulmonary Blood Flow
(Cyanotic: Right-to-left shunt)

A heart defect that features four problems:
- a hole between the ventricles
- aorta lies over the hole in the ventricles
- an obstruction from the heart to the lungs
- right ventricle muscle is thickened

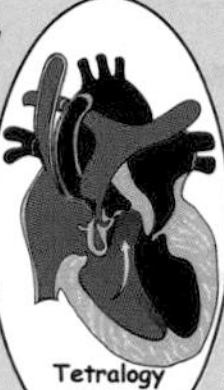

Obstructive Lesions
(No flow)

The narrowed aorta obstructs blood flow from the heart to the lower part of the body.

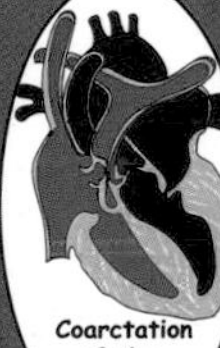

Mixed Lesions
(Caused by blood flow in both directions)

The two main arteries carrying blood away from the heart are reversed.

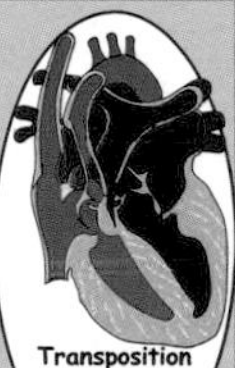

What You Need to Know

Congenital Heart Defects

SIGNIFICANCE OF CONGENITAL HEART DEFECTS

Congenital heart disease is second only to prematurity as a leading cause of death in the first year of life. The underlying cause is unknown. However, genetic factors, the use of some drugs during pregnancy, and prenatal factors all contribute to the development of congenital heart defects.

ANATOMIC DEFECTS

- Valve abnormalities, displaced vessels
- Abnormal openings of the foramen ovale or septum

HEMODYNAMIC CHANGES

- Mixing of pulmonary and systemic blood flow
- Increased or decreased blood flow through pulmonary or systemic circulation
  - Right-to-left shunt—movement of unoxygenated blood to systemic circulation
  - Left-to-right shunt—increased pulmonary blood flow and congestion in pulmonary circulation

DEFECTS DECREASING PULMONARY BLOOD FLOW

- Results in a right-to-left shunt, unoxygenated blood is pumped into left ventricle with decreased blood pumped into the pulmonary artery.
  - Examples: tetralogy of Fallot, tricuspid atresia.
  - Patients are cyanotic and hypoxemic, pulmonary blood flow is low, and congestive heart failure *does not* commonly occur.

DEFECTS INCREASING PULMONARY BLOOD FLOW

- Results in left-to-right shunt, oxygenated blood is returned again to the pulmonary circulation.
  - Examples: patent ductus arteriosus, atrial septal defect, ventricular septal defect.
  - Patients will develop congestive heart failure as a result of increased pulmonary artery blood flow.

MIXED DEFECTS

- Survival depends on additional cardiac defects that allow for the mixing of blood from the pulmonary system and the systemic circulation.
    - Transposition of great vessels—atrial septal defect may provide mixing of blood.
    - Truncus arteriosus—ventricular defect provides for mixing of blood.
    - Pulmonary congestion occurs, and the patient frequently develops congestive heart failure.

Important nursing implications	Serious/life-threatening implications
Most frequent side effects	Patient teaching

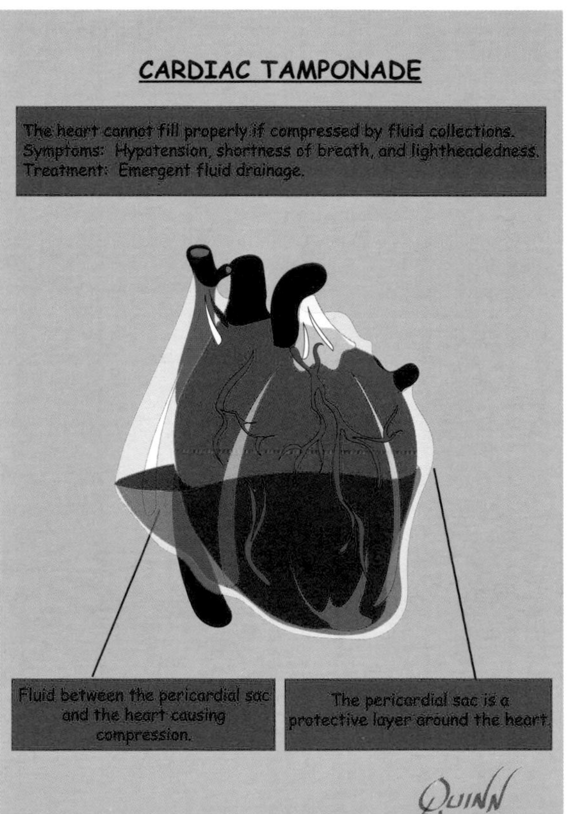
CARDIAC TAMPONADE
The heart cannot fill properly if compressed by fluid collections.
Symptoms: Hypotension, shortness of breath, and lightheadedness.
Treatment: Emergent fluid drainage.
Fluid between the pericardial sac and the heart causing compression.
The pericardial sac is a protective layer around the heart.
Quinn

What You Need to Know

Cardiac Tamponade

SIGNIFICANCE OF CARDIAC TAMPONADE

Cardiac tamponade develops as a result of a pericardial effusion or fluid accumulation in the pericardial sac. Pericardial effusion is most often a complication of pericarditis, but it may occur after coronary artery bypass surgery. The fluid accumulation in the pericardial sac causes a decrease in the atrial and ventricular filling, precipitating a significant decrease in CO. Cardiac tamponade may gradually occur or become an acute problem.

SIGNS AND SYMPTOMS

- Anxiety, restlessness, dizziness
- Pulsus paradoxus—drop in BP on inspiration (decrease is usually greater than 10 mm Hg pressure)
- Presence of JVD
- Muffled heart sounds
- Narrowing pulse pressure
- Tachycardia; hypotension; tachypnea
- Evidence of decreasing CO

MEDICAL TREATMENT

Pericardiocentesis—aspiration of excess pericardial fluid.

Acute cardiac tamponade is an emergency situation that must be immediately addressed.

NURSING MANAGEMENT

- Maintain bedrest and provide oxygen.
- Monitor for dysrhythmias.
- Monitor for further changes in vital signs.
- Maintain patent vascular access line.
- Assess for problems of inadequate tissue perfusion.
- Reassure the patient that the problem is being addressed.

Important nursing implications

Serious/life-threatening implications

Most frequent side effects

Patient teaching

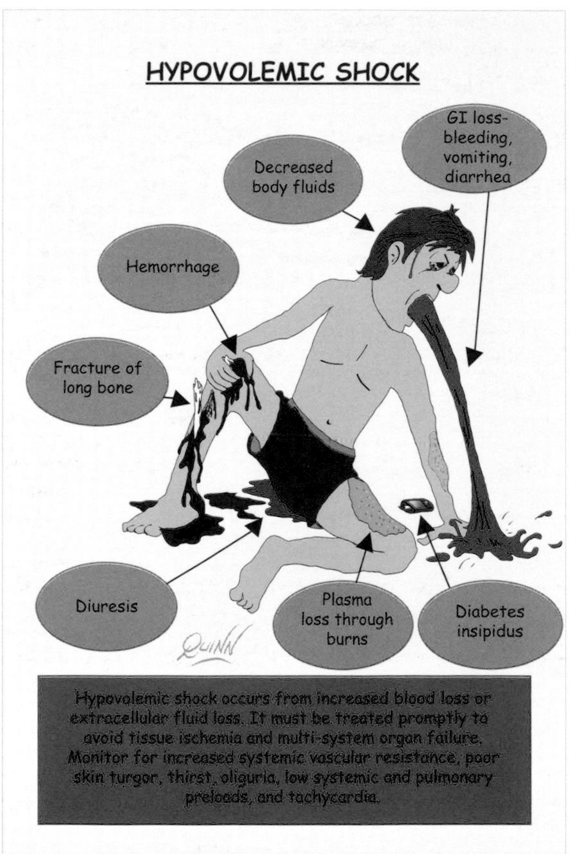
HYPOVOLEMIC SHOCK
GI loss-
bleeding,
vomiting,
diarrhea
Decreased
body fluids
Hemorrhage
Fracture of
long bone
Diuresis
Plasma
loss through
burns
Diabetes
insipidus
QUINN
Hypovolemic shock occurs from increased blood loss or extracellular fluid loss. It must be treated promptly to avoid tissue ischemia and multi-system organ failure. Monitor for increased systemic vascular resistance, poor skin turgor, thirst, oliguria, low systemic and pulmonary preloads, and tachycardia.

What You Need to Know

Hypovolemic Shock

SIGNIFICANCE OF HYPOVOLEMIC SHOCK

Hypovolemic shock is caused by a loss of blood (hemorrhage), plasma (burns), or interstitial fluid (diaphoresis, diabetes insipidus, emesis, or diuresis).

PRECIPITATING FACTORS

Absolute Hypovolemia

- Loss of whole blood (hemorrhage from trauma, surgery, gastrointestinal bleeding)
- Loss of plasma (burn injuries)
- Loss of other body fluids (vomiting, diarrhea, excessive diuresis, diabetes insipidus)

Relative Hypovolemia

- Pooling of blood or fluids (third spacing—ascites, bowel obstruction, peritonitis)
- Internal bleeding (fracture of the long bones, ruptured spleen, hemothorax, severe pancreatitis)
- Massive vasodilation (sepsis)

SIGNS AND SYMPTOMS

- Size of vascular compartment remains unchanged while the volume of blood or plasma decreases, resulting in decreased venous return to the heart, as well as decreased preload, SV, and CO.
- Continuous or further loss of blood volume occurs, which leads to a stimulation of a sympathetic nervous system response.
- HR, CO, and respiratory rate and depth increase in patients who can effectively compensate.
- SV and pulmonary artery wedge pressure decrease as a result of the low-circulating blood volume.
- Decreased urinary output caused by a decrease in renal blood flow resulting in sodium and water retention.

DIAGNOSTIC FINDINGS

- Laboratory tests to evaluate hypovolemic shock include: hemoglobin, hematocrit, urine-specific gravity, electrolytes, and lactate.

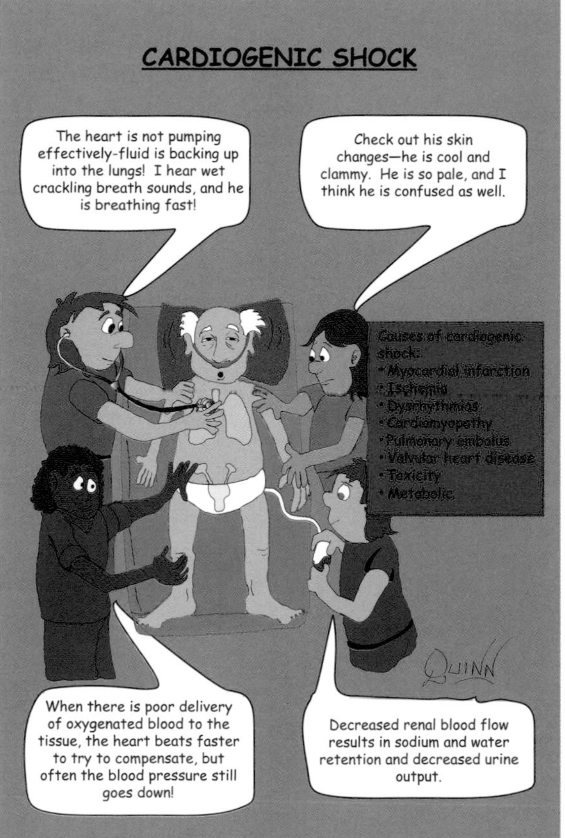
CARDIOGENIC SHOCK
The heart is not pumping effectively-fluid is backing up into the lungs! I hear wet crackling breath sounds, and he is breathing fast!
Check out his skin changes—he is cool and clammy. He is so pale, and I think he is confused as well.
Causes of cardiogenic shock:
• Myocardial infarction
• Ischemia
• Dysrhythmias
• Cardiomyopathy
• Pulmonary embolus
• Valvular heart disease
• Toxicity
• Metabolic
QUINN
When there is poor delivery of oxygenated blood to the tissue, the heart beats faster to try to compensate, but often the blood pressure still goes down!
Decreased renal blood flow results in sodium and water retention and decreased urine output.

What You Need to Know

Cardiogenic Shock

SIGNIFICANCE OF CARDIOGENIC SHOCK

Cardiogenic shock most commonly follows heart failure when either systolic or diastolic dysfunction of the myocardium leads to compromised CO. The patient experiences impaired tissue perfusion, which causes cellular hypoxia throughout the body.

PRECIPITATING FACTORS

- Systolic dysfunction (MI, cardiomyopathy)—inability of the heart to pump blood forward
- Diastolic dysfunction (cardiac tamponade)—inability of the heart to fill during diastole
- Arrhythmias (bradycardia, tachycardia)
- Structural problems—valvular stenosis or regurgitation, acute ventricular septal defect

SIGNS AND SYMPTOMS

- Impaired mentation, anxiety, and delirium; impaired cerebral perfusion
- Tachycardia, increased preload, decreased SV
- Peripheral vasoconstriction, which increases afterload
- Pulmonary congestion, bibasilar crackles, dyspnea, dusky skin color, hypoxemia
- Increased level of CO_2 leading to respiratory acidosis
- Decreased BP, narrow pulse pressure
- Decreased renal blood flow, leading to sodium and water retention; decreased urine output, leading to oliguria
- Precipitates multiple organ dysfunction syndrome (MODS)

DIAGNOSTIC FINDINGS

- Laboratory tests to evaluate cardiogenic shock include: cardiac enzymes, troponin level, electrocardiogram, chest X-ray studies, echocardiogram, and lactate

---

Important nursing implications | Serious/life-threatening implications

Most frequent side effects | Patient teaching

COMMON HEMATOLOGIC PROBLEMS

- Fatigue
- Weak
- Shortness of breath

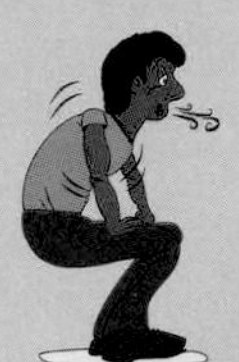

Deficiency of red blood cells will result in decreased hemoglobin, which causes anemia. This will decrease oxygen-carrying capacity of the blood.

Alterations in leukocyte functions can show up in the body's immune and inflammatory responses.

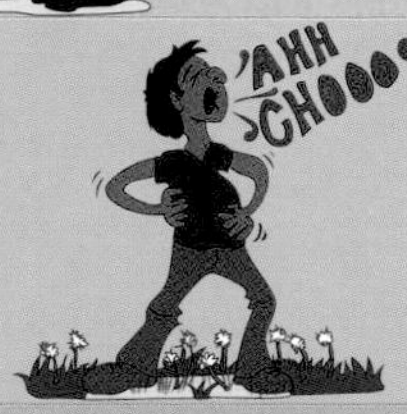

- Itching
- Sneezing
- Inflammation
- Infection

- Bleeding from the nose
- Bleeding from the gums
- Bruising

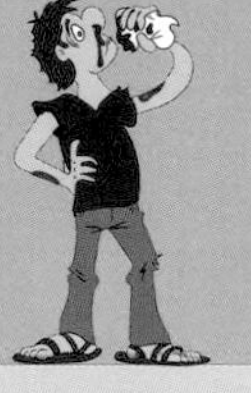

Alterations in platelets and coagulation disorders can cause internal or external hemorrhaging and bruising. Bleeding problems may be caused by medications, bone marrow suppression, or hematologic conditions.

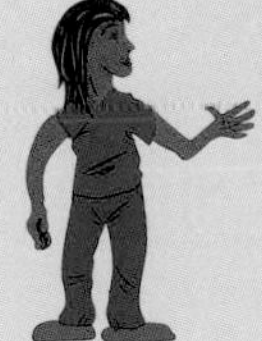

Assessment skills will help the nurse spot these types of conditions and assist the patient before the disorders become more serious or life threatening.

QUINN

What You Need to Know

Common Hematologic Problems

ANEMIA

Anemia can be caused by a deficiency in the number of red blood cells (RBCs) or in the quality and amount of the hemoglobin. A low hemoglobin level decreases the oxygen-carrying capacity of the blood to the tissues. There are many forms of anemia including: aplastic, iron deficiency, sickle cell, thalassemia, and vitamin deficiency.

Causes

- Decreased RBC count (erythrocyte production)
- Loss of blood, acute or chronic
- Increased destruction of RBCs
- Decreased renal production of erythropoietin
- Poor nutrition—decreased intake of iron and vitamin B
- Chemotherapy medications

LEUKOPENIA

Leukopenia is a decrease in the total number of white blood cells (WBCs).

Causes

- Medications, especially chemotherapeutic drugs
- Hematologic problems that cause destruction of WBCs (e.g., leukemia)
- Disease processes and infections—human immunodeficiency virus (HIV), sepsis
- Autoimmune conditions—systemic lupus erythematous, rheumatoid arthritis

PLATELETS, COAGULATION, AND VASCULAR RESPONSE

The process of hemostasis or clotting is initiated by:

- When a vessel is injured, platelets form a plug and begin activation of the coagulation response.
- Coagulation is triggered by intrinsic factors (factors within the blood) or extrinsic factors (factors in response to changes in the blood vessels).
- Thrombin initiates the fibrinogen to form fibrin in clot formation.

Causes

- Increased platelets and coagulation in response to a blood vessel injury
- Decreased platelets (thrombocytopenia)
- Aging—decreased production of thrombocytes by the bone marrow
- Decreased clotting factors—hemophilia
- Response to medications and herbs—aspirin, nonsteroidal antiinflammatory drugs (NSAIDs), vitamin E, *Gingko biloba*, and ginseng

---

Important nursing implications

Serious/life-threatening implications

Most frequent side effects

Patient teaching

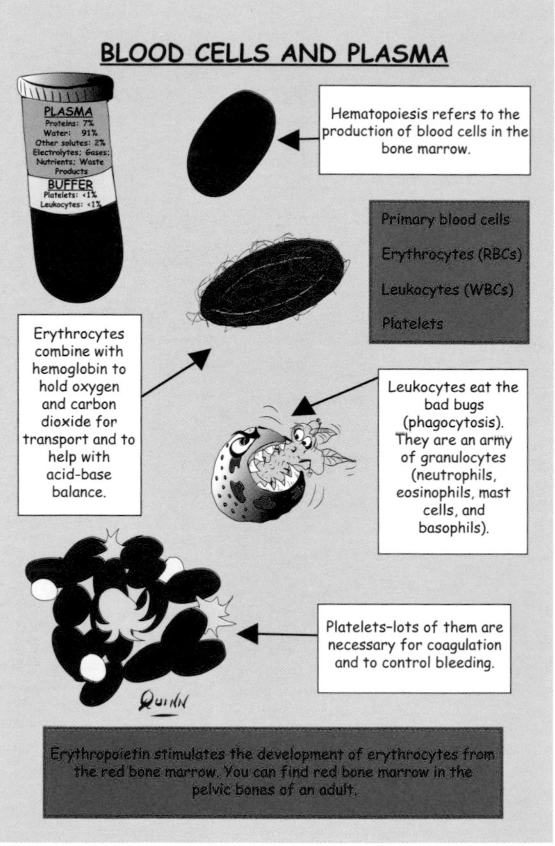
BLOOD CELLS AND PLASMA
PLASMA
Proteins: 7%
Water: 91%
Other solutes: 2%
Electrolytes; Gases;
Nutrients; Waste
Products
BUFFER
Platelets: <1%
Leukocytes: <1%
Hematopoiesis refers to the production of blood cells in the bone marrow.
Primary blood cells
Erythrocytes (RBCs)
Leukocytes (WBCs)
Platelets
Erythrocytes combine with hemoglobin to hold oxygen and carbon dioxide for transport and to help with acid-base balance.
Leukocytes eat the bad bugs (phagocytosis). They are an army of granulocytes (neutrophils, eosinophils, mast cells, and basophils).
Platelets-lots of them are necessary for coagulation and to control bleeding.
QUINN
Erythropoietin stimulates the development of erythrocytes from the red bone marrow. You can find red bone marrow in the pelvic bones of an adult.

What You Need to Know

Blood Cells and Plasma

COMPONENTS OF BLOOD

Blood consists of fluid, cells, and protein that circulate throughout the body via the vascular system. Approximately 5.5 L (6 quarts) of blood circulate in the healthy adult. Electrically charged particles (electrolytes) and proteins maintain the osmolarity and acid-base balance of the blood.

HEMATOPOIESIS

Hematopoiesis refers to the production of blood cells in the bone marrow. It continues throughout life as old blood cells are removed from apoptosis, aging, blood loss through hemorrhage, or as cells are destroyed from diseases.

FUNCTIONS OF BLOOD

- Transports nutrition (protein, glucose, carbohydrates, lipids, vitamins) to the cells.
- Transports oxygen for cellular metabolism. Oxygen is bound to the hemoglobin to form oxyhemoglobin in the RBCs.
- Removes the byproducts of cellular metabolism.
- Carries cells and antibodies that protect the body against infection and invading organisms.

PLASMA

Plasma makes up approximately 55%–60% of the blood volume. Plasma proteins are the primary element, but plasma also contains electrolytes and cellular nutrition.

PLASMA PROTEINS

- *Albumin*—maintains the colloid pressure in the capillaries and arterioles; regulates the movement or passage of water and solutes through the microcirculation.
- *Clotting factors*—initiate the clotting process when vessels have been injured.
- *Lipoproteins*—include triglycerides, cholesterol, and fatty acids.

CELLULAR COMPONENTS

- *Erythrocytes*—are RBCs that contain hemoglobin for oxygen transport.
- *Leukocytes*—are WBCs that defend the body against infection or foreign invasion.
- *Platelets*—are the smallest of the cells. Approximately one-third are stored in the spleen and are the first to respond when a vessel injury occurs to control bleeding through coagulation.

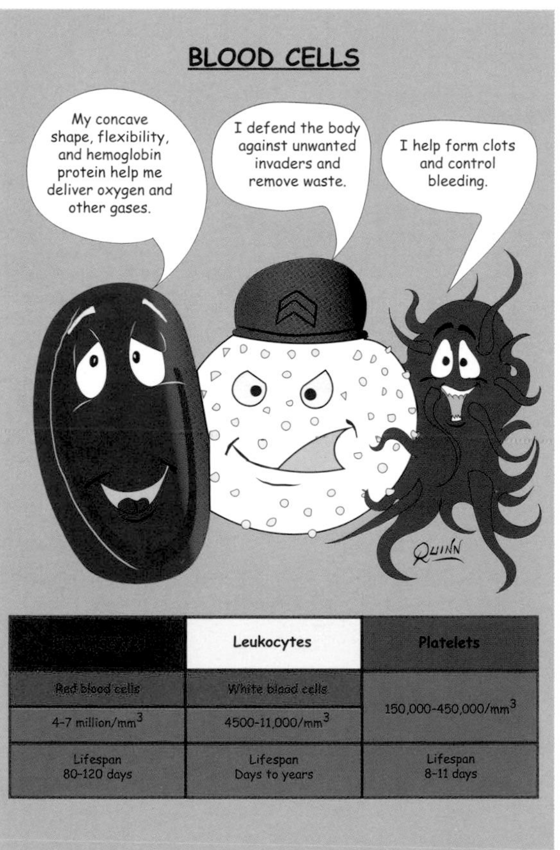

[illegible]	Leukocytes	Platelets
Red blood cells	White blood cells	$150,000-450,000/mm^3$
$4-7$ million$/mm^3$	$4500-11,000/mm^3$	
Lifespan 80-120 days	Lifespan Days to years	Lifespan 8-11 days

What You Need to Know

Blood Cells

SIGNIFICANCE OF ERYTHROCYTES

RBCs are produced by the bone marrow, a process called erythropoiesis. Erythrocytes are RBCs that contain hemoglobin. Hemoglobin is the oxygen-carrying protein in the cell. When oxygen is attached, the blood cell is called *oxyhemoglobin*. Hemoglobin also assists in maintaining acid-base balance of the blood.

Production

- RBCs are produced by the bone marrow.
- The production process is controlled by the level of oxygen in the circulating blood and erythropoietin, which is a hormone from the kidneys.
- Adequate serum levels of iron, vitamin B_{12}, and folic acid are necessary for normal RBC production.
- Normal RBC count: $4–7 \times 10^6$/mcL; hemoglobin: 12–18 g/dL

SIGNIFICANCE OF LEUKOCYTES

WBCs are produced from within the bone marrow and are responsible for fighting infection and for responding to the invasion by foreign cells. They are differentiated.

Production

- WBCs are transported by the blood and defend the body against infection at the tissue level. They are differentiated into two categories: (1) granulocytes (neutrophils, eosinophils, basophils), and (2) agranulocytes (lymphocytes, monocytes).
- Normal total WBC count: 4500–11,000/mm^3

SIGNIFICANCE OF PLATELETS

Platelets are activated when a blood vessel is injured and collagen is released. The platelets clump together and form the platelet plug. The platelet lipoprotein stimulates the beginning of the clotting process and the activation of the clotting factors.

Production

- Platelets are produced in the bone marrow and stored in the spleen where they are slowly released.
- Normal platelet count: 150,000–450,000/mm^3

Important nursing implications

Serious/life-threatening implications

Most frequent side effects

Patient teaching

ABO BLOOD GROUPING

Antigens The presence determines the blood type and Rh factor.	**Blood Types** A,B,AB, and O	**Antibodies** A and B antibodies

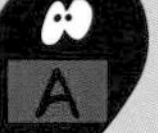
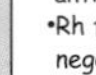

- Type A blood has only the A antigen on red cells and B antibodies in the plasma.
- Rh factor can be positive or negative.

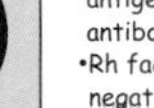

- Type B blood has only the B antigen on red cells and A antibodies in the plasma.
- Rh factor can be positive or negative.

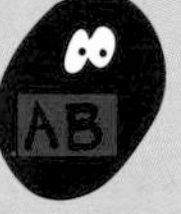

- Type AB blood has both A and B antigens on red cells, but neither A nor B antibodies in the plasma.
- Rh factor can be positive or negative.
- AB positive blood type is a universal recipient-no antibodies against A, B, AB, O, or Rh factor.

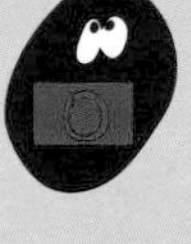

- Type O blood has neither A nor B antigens on red cells, but has both A and B antibodies in the plasma.
- Rh factor can be positive or negative.
- O negative blood type is a universal donor but cannot accept blood from an A, B, AB, or Rh positive donor.

- Rh positive or Rh negative blood is based on the presence or absense of the D-antigen.
- Rh negative donor may be transfused to all blood types (factor is absent).
- Rh positive donor must be transfused only to Rh positive recipients (factor is present).

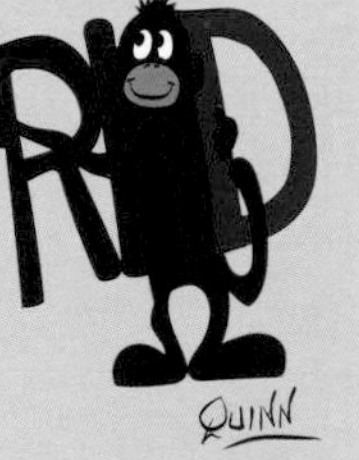

What You Need to Know

ABO Blood Grouping

SIGNIFICANCE OF BLOOD GROUPING AND THE RH FACTOR

- RBCs (erythrocytes) are grouped according to types A, B, and O. Four blood types are possible—A, B, AB, and O. Type A blood has antibodies for type B; type B blood has antibodies for type A. Type AB blood has no antibodies for A or B blood type. Type O blood has both type A and B antibodies.
- When a serum antibody reacts with the antigen on the RBC membrane, the process will result in hemolysis of the erythrocyte. Hemolysis will occur if a patient with type A blood is given a transfusion from a donor with type B blood. Type A blood has only A antigen. Type B blood has B antigen. Type AB blood has both A and B antigens. Type O blood has neither type A nor B antigens. Rh factor (D-antigen) is present in the blood of a person who is Rh positive (+) and is not present in Rh negative (–) blood.
- O negative blood is identified as the *universal donor*, but cannot accept blood from an A, B, AB, or Rh positive donor. **O negative blood is transfused to patients with type A, B, or AB only in extreme emergencies.**
- The patient with AB positive blood is considered the *universal recipient*, the Rh factor (D-antigen) is present, and both A and B antigens are present. **Patients with AB positive blood can receive type A, B, or AB blood, but only in extreme emergencies.**

IMPLICATIONS FOR NURSING

- When a pregnant woman is Rh– and carrying a fetus that is Rh+, the woman may develop antibodies against the Rh+ fetus.
- Rho(D) immune globulin is given to prevent (or protect) the development of the Rh antibodies that would affect subsequent pregnancies.

Important nursing implications | Serious/life-threatening implications

Most frequent side effects | Patient teaching

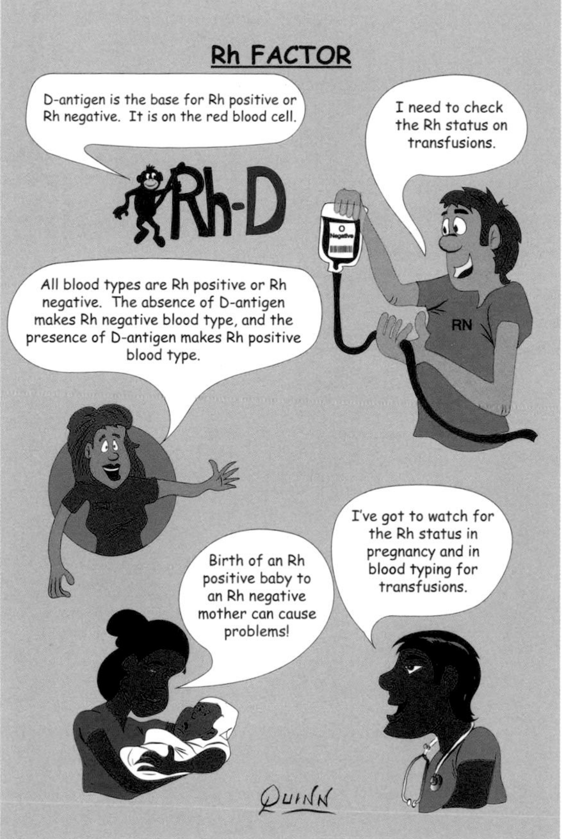
Rh FACTOR
D-antigen is the base for Rh positive or Rh negative. It is on the red blood cell.
Rh-D
I need to check the Rh status on transfusions.
O Negative
RN
All blood types are Rh positive or Rh negative. The absence of D-antigen makes Rh negative blood type, and the presence of D-antigen makes Rh positive blood type.
Birth of an Rh positive baby to an Rh negative mother can cause problems!
I've got to watch for the Rh status in pregnancy and in blood typing for transfusions.
QUINN

What You Need to Know

Rh Factor

SIGNIFICANCE OF THE RH FACTOR

The RhD protein is a dominant antigen on the erythrocytes. The presence of the antigen makes a person Rh+ and the absence of the antigen is Rh–. The presence or absence of the antigen in an individual has implications in the administration of blood and in pregnancy.

Blood Transfusions

- Before administering blood, the recipient's blood must be crossmatched for the presence of the Rh antigen. The donor blood is also crossmatched for compatibility with the recipient's blood.
- An individual who is Rh+ may receive donor blood from a person who is Rh– because the antigen is not present in the donor's blood. However, a person who is Rh– cannot receive Rh+ donor blood because of the presence of the Rh antigen.

Rh Factor and Pregnancy

- If a woman is Rh– and is pregnant with an Rh+ infant, she will develop antibodies against the Rh antigen.
- To prevent the development of the antibodies or sensitization, the mother will receive the Rh immune globulin (RhoGAM) after delivery to suppress the immune response and to prevent the development of Rh antibodies.
- Rh– women should receive RhoGAM between 20 and 30 weeks gestation or after birth and after a miscarriage or ectopic pregnancy in which the possibility of sensitization with Rh+ antigens exists.
- A current pregnancy or exposure is not a problem; however, a future pregnancy with an Rh+ infant would cause the destruction of fetal erythrocytes and result in hemolytic disease in the newborn.

Infant

- Infants should never receive the RhoGAM.
- In the first pregnancy, the infant is not affected.
- In future pregnancies with an Rh+ fetus, the mother may have been sensitized against the Rh antibodies, and destruction of the fetal erythrocytes will affect the Rh+ fetus.
- RhoGam is administered to the mother in the first and subsequent pregnancies to prevent this sensitization.

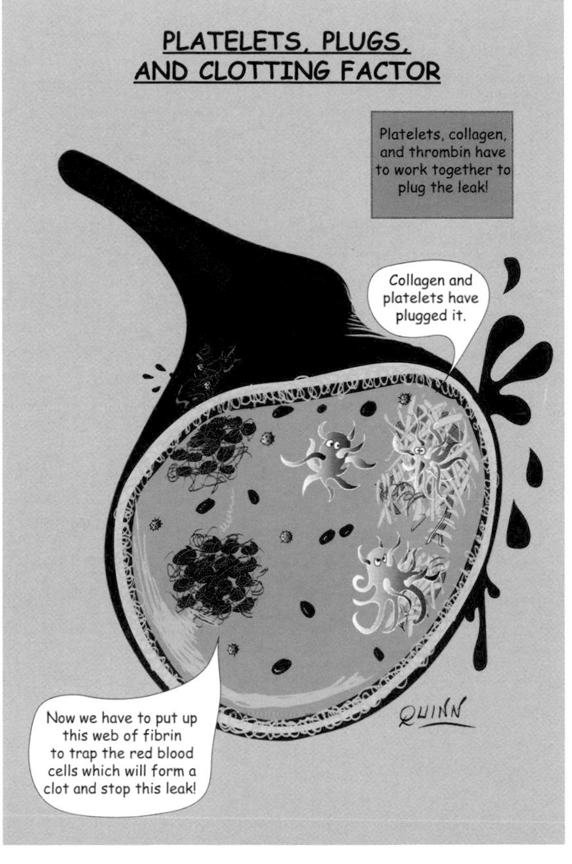
PLATELETS, PLUGS, AND CLOTTING FACTOR
Platelets, collagen, and thrombin have to work together to plug the leak!
Collagen and platelets have plugged it.
Now we have to put up this web of fibrin to trap the red blood cells which will form a clot and stop this leak!
QUINN

What You Need to Know

Platelets, Plugs, and Clotting Factors

FACTORS OF CLOTTING

- *Intrinsic factors*—include problems or substances in the blood that make the platelets clump and activate the clotting cascade.
- *Extrinsic factors*—include activity outside the cell that damages a blood vessel and exposes platelets to collagen and activates the clotting cascade.

PLATELETS

- Normally circulate in plasma. Collagen from a damaged vessel activates the platelets.
- Platelet membranes become rough and sticky, promoting the adhesion of the platelets and the development of the platelet plug.
- Platelet plug is not a clot, but it initiates the activation of the clotting cascade. Platelet aggregation is facilitated by the presence of fibrinogen, which traps more RBCs and debris to form a clot.

CLOTTING CASCADE

- Clotting cascade—is a series of steps that begins with the fibrinogen conversion to prothrombin, then to thromboplastin, and on through the series of coagulation steps or factors to form a clot.
- Regardless of the cause of the injury, the clotting functions continue to follow the same common pathway—the aggregation of the platelets, the deposition of the fibrin at the injured site, and the collection of the RBCs to form the clot.
- At each step, the activated enzyme from the previous level initiates the action of the next level.

CLOT RETRACTION

- After the initiation and completion of the steps in the formation of a clot, a control factor must limit the activity.
- Once a clot has formed, the fibrin strands absorb the thrombin produced at the site.
- Clot begins to retract or solidify in the final stage of hemostasis.
- Fibrinolysin splits fibrin and fibrinogen into degradation products that will dissolve the clot.

Important nursing implications | Serious/life-threatening implications
Most frequent side effects | Patient teaching

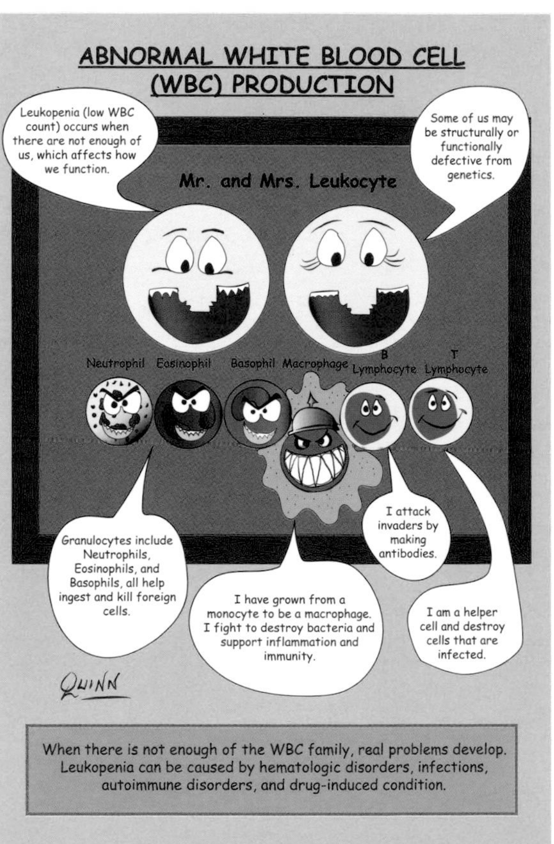
ABNORMAL WHITE BLOOD CELL (WBC) PRODUCTION
Leukopenia (low WBC count) occurs when there are not enough of us, which affects how we function.
Some of us may be structurally or functionally defective from genetics.
Mr. and Mrs. Leukocyte
Neutrophil
Eosinophil
Basophil
Macrophage
B Lymphocyte
T Lymphocyte
I attack invaders by making antibodies.
Granulocytes include Neutrophils, Eosinophils, and Basophils, all help ingest and kill foreign cells.
I have grown from a monocyte to be a macrophage. I fight to destroy bacteria and support inflammation and immunity.
I am a helper cell and destroy cells that are infected.
QUINN
When there is not enough of the WBC family, real problems develop. Leukopenia can be caused by hematologic disorders, infections, autoimmune disorders, and drug-induced condition.

What You Need to Know

Abnormal White Blood Cell Production

SIGNIFICANCE OF ABNORMAL WBC PRODUCTION

WBCs protect the body from infection and maintain a normal immune system. The normal body's defense mechanisms are affected when any type of the WBC is present in elevated or decreased numbers.

TYPES OF WBCS

- *Granulocytes* (neutrophils, eosinophils, basophils)—make up the largest group of leukocytes. These mature cells are the first line of defense against invading organisms. The more granulocytes that are present, the better the defense. Cell count is high with infection and inflammation.
- *Monocytes* (macrophages)—are strong phagocytes and ingest dead or defective cells. Migration out of the bone marrow occurs in response to infection or inflammation. Monocytes are the primary cells involved in the beginning stages of inflammation. They initiate the process that allows B and T cells to recognize the antigens (foreign agents).
- *B lymphocytes and T lymphocytes*—B lymphocytes are developed in the bone marrow, whereas T lymphocytes are processed through the thymus. B cells are responsible for producing antibodies and are important in humoral immunity. T cells are known as cytotoxic killer or helper T cells. B and T cells work together to recognize a foreign agent or antigen and, along with macrophages, begin to differentiate invading cells from normal body cells. The production of antibodies against an antigen occurs as part of the body's normal immune response.

LEUKOPENIA

- Occurs when an insufficient number of WBCs are present.
  - Too few cells produced
  - Premature destruction of cells
  - Disrupted leukocyte function
- *Causes*—leukopenia occurs with multiple diseases or conditions. The cause may be iatrogenic, a side effect of medications, or a result of chemotherapy medications.
- *Implications*—patient is predisposed to infections that would not normally cause problems (opportunistic infections). Leukopenia may mask the signs of infection such as an elevated white count. A slight elevation in body temperature may be significant in an individual with leukopenia because usually the individual is immunocompromised, and minor infections can develop into major problems.

NEGATVE-FEEDBACK CONTROL OF HORMONES

Endocrine System Negative-Feedback Loops

Negative-feedback systems are important in maintaining hormones within physiologic ranges.

+

The lack of feedback inhibition on hormonal release results in pathologic conditions.

+

Hormonal imbalances and related conditions from excessive hormone production are caused by the inability to turn off.

+

Negative feedback is a system in which plasma levels of one type of hormones influence levels of others.

Negative feedback isn't always a bad thing.

QUINN

What You Need to Know

Negative-Feedback Control of Hormones

SIGNIFICANCE OF CONTROL OF HORMONES

Hormone regulation is mostly done by *negative-feedback control,* which is when a hormone causes an effect on a target gland. When the hormone levels are high, they inhibit the hypothalamus and anterior pituitary gland from secreting those hormones, resulting in a decline in hormone levels.

HOW IT WORKS

- Endocrine glands respond by increasing or decreasing the amount of hormones secreted.
- Hormone secretion is determined by the hormonal levels in the circulatory system.
- Endocrine glands release hormones into the circulatory system.
- Most hormones travel to the target tissue to increase or decrease activity.
- An increase in the secretion of a hormone occurs when low levels of the hormone are in circulation, which causes negative feedback.

Example: Insulin Production

- When blood glucose levels start to rise, the islets of Langerhans in the pancreas are stimulated to secrete insulin.
- When blood glucose levels begin to drop, insulin production decreases.
- Some hormones have a more complex interaction and use the negative-feedback mechanism for interactions among the endocrine glands.

Example: Thyroid Stimulating Hormone (TSH) Production

- TSH comes from the anterior pituitary gland. It responds to low levels of circulating thyroxin. Thyroid hormone thyroxine (T4) is a precursor to triiodothyronine (T3), which regulates the metabolic rate of all the cells and processes of cell growth. Therefore, when a decrease in the circulating levels of the thyroid hormone occurs, the anterior pituitary gland recognizes the need for more thyroid hormone. The anterior pituitary gland sends a signal to the thyroid gland to produce more thyroid hormone. Circulating levels of TSH are used to monitor the thyroid conditions and hormonal levels—when the TSH level is too high, a decrease in or an insufficient level of the circulating thyroid hormone has occurred, and more is needed.
- When a lack of stimulation or inhibition occurs on the control of the endocrine hormones, pathologic disorders will occur.

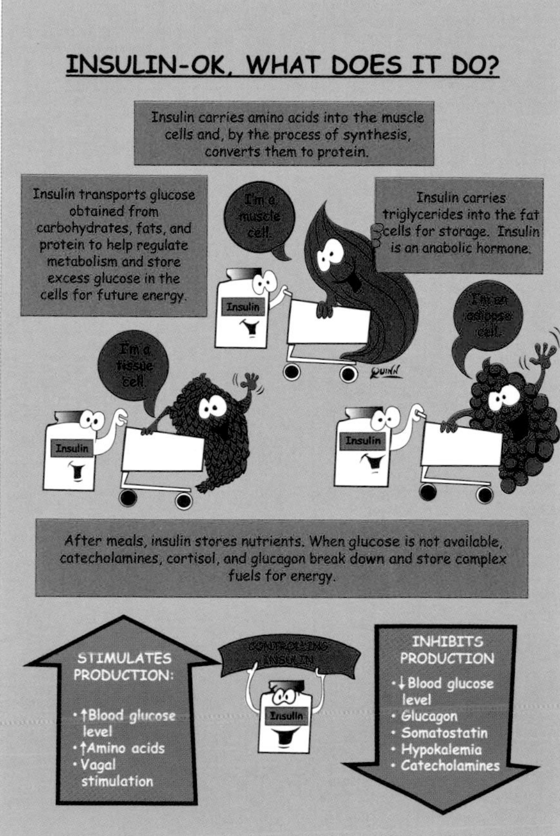
INSULIN-OK, WHAT DOES IT DO?
Insulin carries amino acids into the muscle cells and, by the process of synthesis, converts them to protein.
Insulin transports glucose obtained from carbohydrates, fats, and protein to help regulate metabolism and store excess glucose in the cells for future energy.
I'm a muscle cell.
Insulin carries triglycerides into the fat cells for storage. Insulin is an anabolic hormone.
Insulin
I'm an adipose cell.
I'm a tissue cell.
Insulin
Insulin
After meals, insulin stores nutrients. When glucose is not available, catecholamines, cortisol, and glucagon break down and store complex fuels for energy.
STIMULATES PRODUCTION:
• ↑Blood glucose level
• ↑Amino acids
• Vagal stimulation
CONTROLLING INSULIN
Insulin
INHIBITS PRODUCTION
• ↓Blood glucose level
• Glucagon
• Somatostatin
• Hypokalemia
• Catecholamines

What You Need to Know

Insulin—OK, What Does It Do?

SIGNIFICANCE OF INSULIN PRODUCTION

Insulin functions as an anabolic hormone, which stimulates growth and promotes the movement and storage of carbohydrates, protein, and fat. The primary sites of insulin synthesis are in the liver, muscle, and adipose tissue, which stimulates cellular metabolism. The major effect of insulin release is to decrease blood glucose. When a decrease in the blood glucose occurs, a decrease in the secretion of insulin is the result (negative feedback control).

INSULIN EFFECTS ON THE LIVER

- Inhibits glycogenolysis (catabolism of glycogen to glucose; hormones glucagon and epinephrine stimulate glycogenolysis), gluconeogenesis (formation of glucose from noncarbohydrate sources, such as amino acids and the glycerol portion of fats), and ketogenesis (process by which ketone bodies are produced as a result of fatty acid breakdown).
- Increases glycogen synthesis and storage.
- Increases triglyceride synthesis.

INSULIN EFFECTS ON MUSCLE

- Promotes protein synthesis.
- Increases amino acid transport.
- Promotes glycogenesis (conversion of glucose to glycogen).

INSULIN EFFECTS ON FAT

- Increases fatty acid synthesis.
- Promotes triglyceride storage.
- Decreases lipolysis (breakdown of fat stored in fat cells).

Important nursing implications | Serious/life-threatening implications
Most frequent side effects | Patient teaching

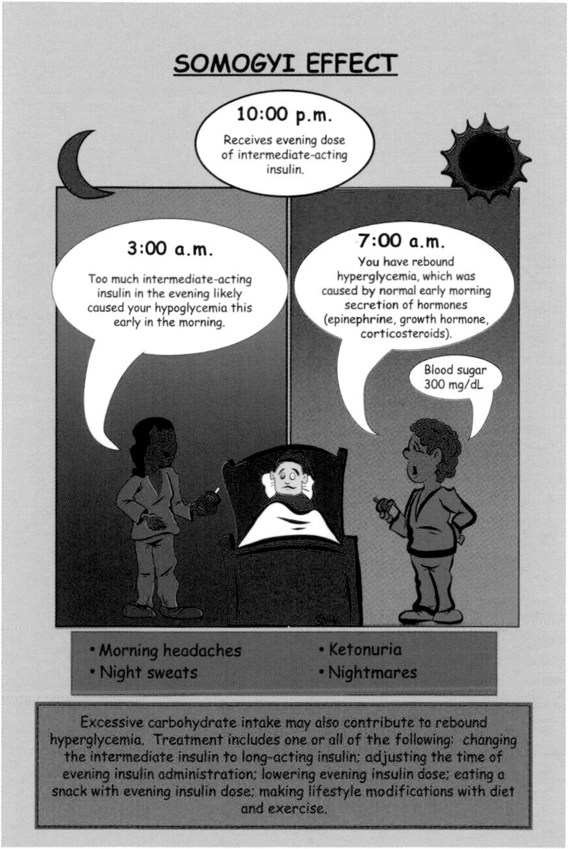

SOMOGYI EFFECT

10:00 p.m.

Receives evening dose of intermediate-acting insulin.

3:00 a.m.

Too much intermediate-acting insulin in the evening likely caused your hypoglycemia this early in the morning.

7:00 a.m.

You have rebound hyperglycemia, which was caused by normal early morning secretion of hormones (epinephrine, growth hormone, corticosteroids).

Blood sugar 300 mg/dL

- Morning headaches
- Night sweats
- Ketonuria
- Nightmares

Excessive carbohydrate intake may also contribute to rebound hyperglycemia. Treatment includes one or all of the following: changing the intermediate insulin to long-acting insulin; adjusting the time of evening insulin administration; lowering evening insulin dose; eating a snack with evening insulin dose; making lifestyle modifications with diet and exercise.

What You Need to Know

Somogyi Effect

SIGNIFICANCE OF THE SOMOGYI EFFECT

The *Somogyi effect* is characterized by wide differences in the blood glucose in the morning (hyperglycemia) and during the night (hypoglycemia) and is associated with undetected episodes of hypoglycemia during sleep.

Morning hyperglycemia may occur because of the counter-regulatory mechanism to the low blood glucose level during the night. The counter-regulatory hormones (epinephrine, cortisol, and glucagon) respond to the low level of blood glucose with an increase in gluconeogenesis and glycogenolysis, which will then produce rebound hyperglycemia.

The problem with the Somogyi effect is that if the blood sugar is high in the morning, then it is often treated with an increase in the insulin dose, which causes worsening of hypoglycemia during the night.

DIAGNOSTICS

- Levels of blood glucose are evaluated by the patient or the nurse during the night (2, 4, 6 a.m.) to confirm the presence of hypoglycemia.

SIGNS AND SYMPTOMS

- Individual may complain of night sweats, morning headaches, or nightmares, which are symptoms of hypoglycemia. Individual may also have ketonuria.

CORRECTION OF THE PROBLEM

- Increase complex carbohydrate intake at bedtime; decrease simple carbohydrate intake.
- Evaluate the type and amount of insulin administered at bedtime. Decrease the insulin affecting the early morning blood glucose.
- Evaluate patient diet, exercise and overall glucose control.
- Teach the patient the importance of evaluating blood glucose levels during the night for several nights to identify the trend.

Important nursing implications
Serious/life-threatening implications
Most frequent side effects
Patient teaching

DAWN PHENOMENON

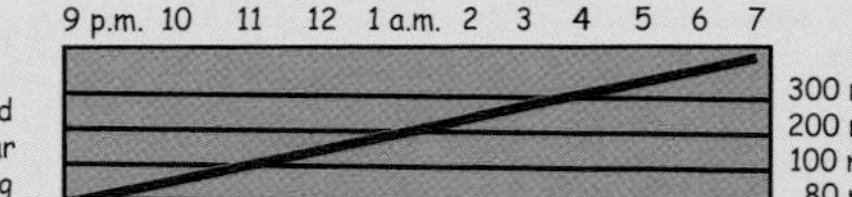

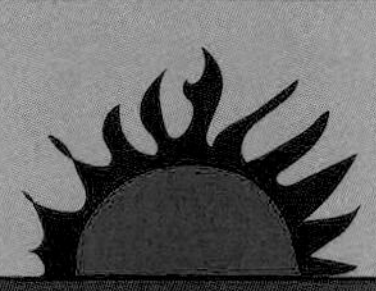

Hyperglycemia in early morning is due to the night time release of the growth hormone-no hypoglycemia during the night.

The dawn phenomenon can affect anyone with diabetes, but it is most severe when the growth hormone is peaking in adolescents and young adults. The growth hormone decreases peripheral glucose uptake and may also be associated with increased clearance of plasma insulin.

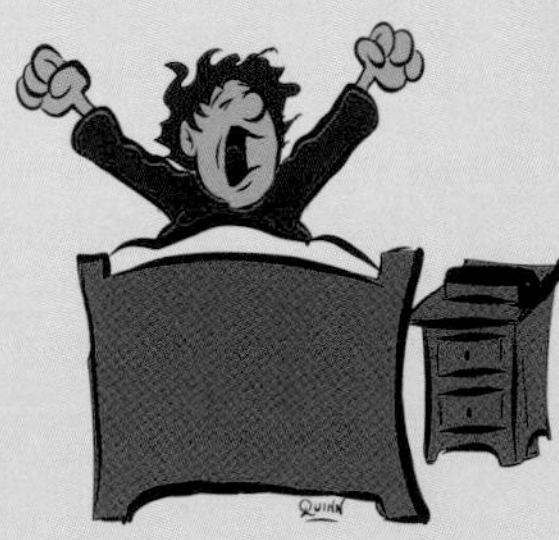

Treatment includes eating a protein snack at bedtime and limiting the intake of carbohydrates and/or increasing the dose of evening insulin.

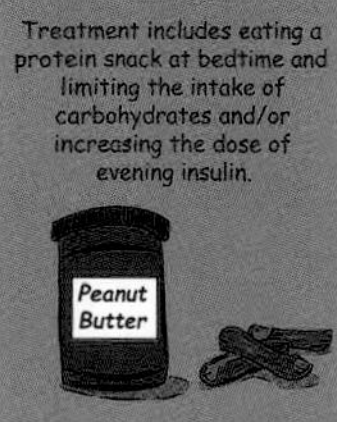

What You Need to Know

Dawn Phenomenon

SIGNIFICANCE OF DAWN PHENOMENON

The *dawn phenomenon* occurs with an increased level of blood glucose during the early morning hours and is not associated with hypoglycemia during the night. Theoretically, the release of the growth hormone during the night causes blood glucose to elevate in the early morning hours at approximately 5–7 a.m. The growth hormone is a counter-regulatory hormone that produces hyperglycemia by decreasing peripheral uptake of glucose.

This phenomenon affects most patients with diabetes, but it tends to be most severe when it is associated with adolescents and young adults with diabetes when the growth hormone level is at a peak.

DIAGNOSTICS

- Evaluate blood glucose levels during the night to differentiate the problem from the Somogyi effect.
- Patients should document the glucose level at bedtime, during the night (2 and 4 a.m.), and in the morning for a fasting level. Several nights should be monitored to validate the trend.

CORRECTION OF THE PROBLEM

- Increase the insulin or adjust the timing of the nighttime insulin dose (given at 10 p.m.).
- If the predawn levels are below 60 mg/dL and the patient is showing signs of hypoglycemia, then reduce the insulin dose.
- If the 2 and 4 a.m. glucose levels are high, then increase the insulin dose.
- Encourage a protein snack at bedtime, and limit the intake of carbohydrates.

Important nursing implications	Serious/life-threatening implications
Most frequent side effects	Patient teaching

CUSHING SYNDROME

When I get hyperfunctional, I can secrete either cortisol or adrenocorticotropic hormones (ACTH) or both. These increased levels can be destructive to the health of the body.

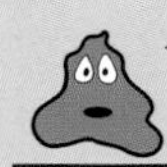

Adrenal gland

Treatment is cause-specific and may consist of medication, radiation or surgery.

Moon face

Sodium and water retention

Slow wound healing

Muscle wasting–thin extremities

Increased BP

Hypokalemia

Truncal obesity

Purple striae

Peptic ulcers

Osteoporosis

Polyuria

Remember, patients who are taking moderate-to-high doses of steroids for chronic inflammatory disorders may also develop Cushing-like symptoms.

What You Need to Know

Cushing Syndrome

SIGNIFICANCE OF CUSHING SYNDROME

Hypercortisolism (adrenocortical hyperfunction) is a condition that is the result of excess levels of adrenal cortex hormones (primarily glucocorticoids) and, to a lesser extent, androgen and aldosterone. Long-term steroid therapy (iatrogenic) is most often the cause of Cushing syndrome.

SIGNS AND SYMPTOMS

- Changes in appearance—characteristic fat deposit, moon face, buffalo hump, truncal obesity with thin extremities, thin skin, purple striae, bruises, and petechiae
- Significant change in personality, and hypertension
- Gastrointestinal (GI) distress (peptic ulcer) from increased acid production; osteoporosis; increased susceptibility to infection, and fluid retention
- Changes in secondary sexual characteristics—amenorrhea (women), hirsutism (women), and gynecomastia (men)
- Diagnostic tests reveal—increased serum sodium, decreased serum potassium hyperglycemia (persistent), increased plasma cortisol levels, loss of diurnal variation of cortisone levels, dexamethasone suppression test

NURSING IMPLICATIONS

- Restrict sodium and water intake; monitor fluid and electrolyte levels. Because of excessive sodium and water retention, monitor for edema, hypertension, and congestive heart failure.
- Watch for potassium depletion. Monitor for cardiac arrhythmias.
- Evaluate for hyperglycemia.
- Assess for GI disturbances.
- Prevent infection.
- Evaluate the patient's ability to cope with changes in body image.
- Monitor for joint and bone pain.
- Promote weight-bearing activities because of the predisposition to fracture.

Important nursing implications | Serious/life-threatening implications

Most frequent side effects | Patient teaching

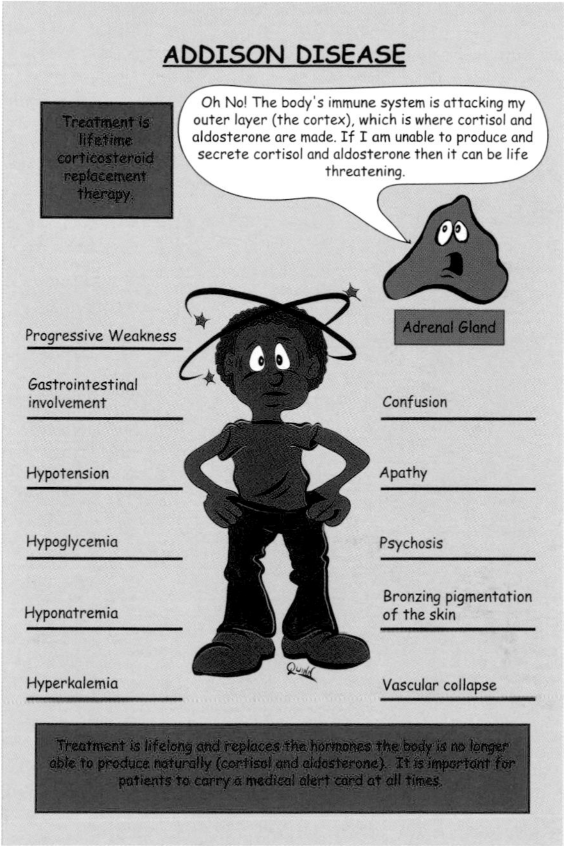

ADDISON DISEASE

Treatment is lifetime corticosteroid replacement therapy.

Oh No! The body's immune system is attacking my outer layer (the cortex), which is where cortisol and aldosterone are made. If I am unable to produce and secrete cortisol and aldosterone then it can be life threatening.

Adrenal Gland

Progressive Weakness

Gastrointestinal involvement

Hypotension

Hypoglycemia

Hyponatremia

Hyperkalemia

Confusion

Apathy

Psychosis

Bronzing pigmentation of the skin

Vascular collapse

QUINN

Treatment is lifelong and replaces the hormones the body is no longer able to produce naturally (cortisol and aldosterone). It is important for patients to carry a medical alert card at all times.

What You Need to Know

Addison Disease

SIGNIFICANCE OF ADDISON DISEASE

Addison disease is an autoimmune-induced disorder caused by a decrease in secretion of the adrenal cortex hormones (cortisol and aldosterone) and is characterized by the following:

- Decreased physiologic response to stress, vascular insufficiency, and hypoglycemia.
- Aldosterone secretions (mineralocorticoids) decrease, which normally promotes a concentration of sodium and water, as well as excretion of potassium.
- Adrenal androgen secretion, which is necessary for secondary sex characteristics, may be altered.
- Occurs after bilateral adrenalectomy or the abrupt withdrawal from long-term corticosteroid therapy.
- Adrenal crisis may be precipitated by a failure of the patient to take medications or increased emotional stress without appropriate hormone replacement.
- Acquired immunodeficiency syndrome (AIDS) and infection are identified as causes of adrenal insufficiency.

SIGNS AND SYMPTOMS

- Development of symptoms requires a loss of 90% of both adrenal cortices.
- Onset is insidious. The patient may or may not have symptoms for weeks to months before diagnosis.
- Fatigue, weakness, weight loss, GI disturbances, bronze pigmentation of the skin, postural hypotension, hyponatremia, hyperkalemia, and hypoglycemia may develop.
- Adrenal crisis—profound fatigue, dehydration, vascular collapse, pallor, anxiety, weak and rapid pulse, tachycardia, and low blood pressure occur.
- Diagnostics—lack of response to adrenocorticotropic hormone (ACTH) stimulation test; decreased serum sodium, increased serum potassium, and decreased cortisol.

TREATMENT

- Replace corticosteroids.
- Life-long steroid therapy is necessary.
- Dose of steroids may need to be increased in times of additional stress.
- Infection, diaphoresis, and injury will necessitate an increase in the need for steroids and may precipitate a crisis state.

AGING AND ENDOCRINE SYSTEM FUNCTION

THE GREAT DEBATE

The relationship between aging and the endocrine system is not clear...

We must be able to recognize if altered endocrine functions are the result of aging...or the cause of aging!
QUINN

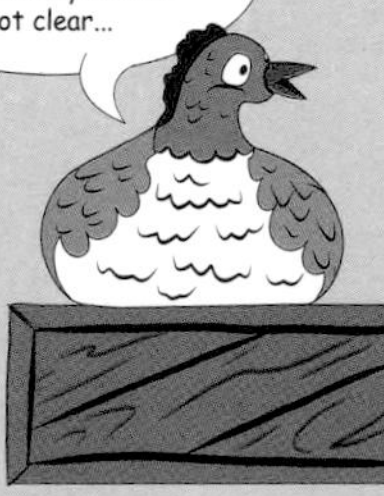

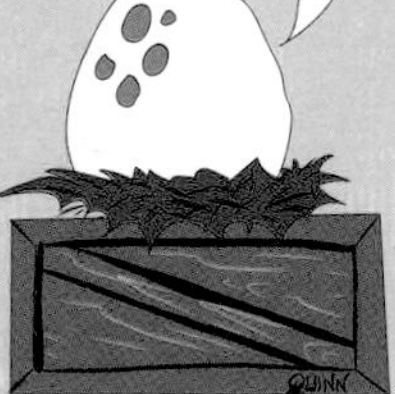

The aging process can alter the production, secretion, and catabolism of hormones. Examples include menopause and the inability to reproduce from a decrease in estrogen, progesterone, and testosterone hormone levels.

What You Need to Know

Aging and Endocrine System Function

SIGNIFICANCE OF AGING AND ENDOCRINE SYSTEM FUNCTION

- Effects of aging on the endocrine system include the following:
  - Decreased hormone production
  - Decreased activity and altered hormone metabolism
  - Changes in circadian rhythms
  - Decreased response of target tissue to hormone changes
- Problems occur when assessing the changes in a patient.
  - Is the assessment finding an anticipated change with the aging process?
  - Is the assessment finding reflective of an endocrine pathology?

NORMAL CHANGES WITH AGING

- **Thyroid**—decreased thyroid function; decreased TSH and T_3
  Assessment: Decreased metabolism may develop, which may cause constipation, lethargy, and mental deterioration.
- **Parathyroid**—increased levels of parathyroid hormone (PTH)
  Assessment: Hypercalcemia, increased bone resorption, and osteoporosis will occur.
- **Adrenal cortex**—increased levels of cortisol; decreased levels of aldosterone
  Assessment: Loss of diurnal and circadian patterns of cortisol secretion, weight gain, protein wasting, and glucose intolerance are evident.
- **Adrenal medulla**—increased levels of norepinephrine; decreased response to beta-adrenergic receptors
  Assessment: Increased fatigue, hypoglycemia, and a lowered response to stress.
- **Pancreas**—increased problems with glucose control; decreased response and sensitivity to insulin
  Assessment: Poor glucose control occurs. Patients with type 2 diabetes are at an increased risk for developing hyperglycemic hyperosmolar nonketoacidosis (HHNK), peripheral neuropathy, changes in major vessels associated with hypertension, and atherosclerotic disease.
- **Gonads**—decreased estrogen secretion in women; decreased testosterone secretion in men

Assessment: Decline in levels of estrogen, which causes problems associated with menopause and results in an increased risk for osteoporosis. Decline in testosterone may not cause problems; however, it can have the effects of decreased sexual function and a loss of bone density and muscle mass.

- **Posterior pituitary**—decreased levels of antidiuretic hormone (ADH)
  Assessment: Maintaining osmolarity of urine becomes difficult. Hyponatremia develops.

Important nursing implications | Serious/life-threatening implications
Most frequent side effects | Patient teaching

COMMON CLUES TO MUSCULOSKELETAL WOES

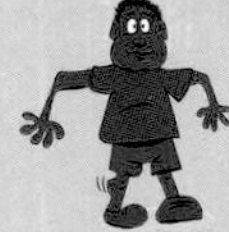

D *Deformity*

Bone or muscle disease, as well as trauma, can cause alterations in bone and muscle shape.

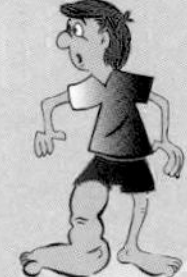

E *Edema*

Fluid that causes edema in the interstitial tissue interferes with nerve function and blood flow, causing tissue deterioration.

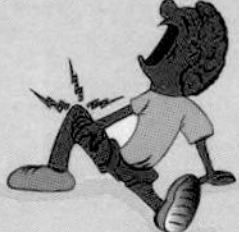

P *Pain*

Pain may occur from pressure on the nerve and/or circulatory compromise.

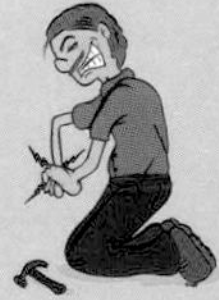

T *Throbbing*

Throbbing occurs as a result of swelling and edema, which further compromises blood supply to the tissues and will slow blood flow.

What You Need to Know

Common Clues to Musculoskeletal Woes

SIGNIFICANCE OF MUSCULOSKELETAL INJURIES

Musculoskeletal injury affects the muscles, bones, joints, ligaments, and tendons. Musculoskeletal trauma accounts for more than half of all injuries and is one of the primary causes of disability.

- Deformity
  - Extremity is out of alignment.
  - Muscle spasm and gravity, as well as the force that caused the injury, determine the position of the bone fracture.
- Edema and swelling around injured area
  - Damage to the soft tissue, bleeding, and inflammation of surrounding tissue will cause pain and may compromise circulation.
  - Compartment syndrome—occurs when an increase in pressure develops within a confined space or compartment of the muscle.
    - Compromises nerve and circulation within the compartment.
    - Treatment must occur within hours to prevent permanent nerve and tissue damage.
    - Increasing pain unrelieved by analgesics is characteristic.
    - Most commonly occurs in injuries to the lower leg and forearm.
    - Pressure in the compartment may be from external pressure (cast) or from internal pressure (bleeding within compartment).
- Pain
  - Occurs immediately in the area of the injury.
  - Subsequent pain may be caused by muscle spasm, overriding of fracture, and further damage to soft tissue in the area.
  - Throbbing pain results as the swelling occurs in the soft tissue and compression of soft tissue and vessels develops.

FIVE Ps OF NEUROVASCULAR COMPROMISE (COMPARTMENT SYNDROME)

- **Paresthesia**—numbness and tingling of extremity
- **Paralysis**—inability to move extremity
- **Pallor**—pale, cool to touch
- **Pain**—unrelieved by medication and out of proportion to injury
- **Pulses**—diminished or absent pulses distal to injury

TYPES OF FRACTURES

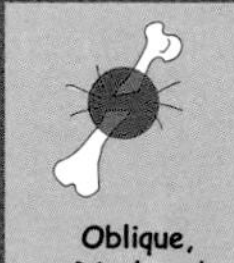

Oblique, Displaced

Sloped or curved break, bone ends ARE NOT aligned

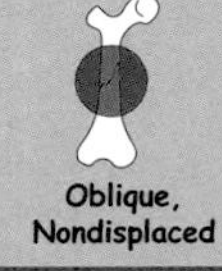

Oblique, Nondisplaced

Sloped or curved break, bone ends ARE aligned

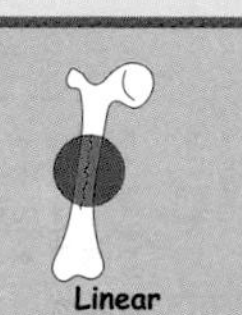

Linear

Break parallel to long axis of bone

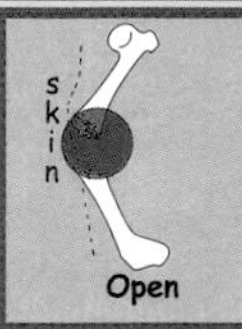

Open

Fragment of bone protruding through an open wound

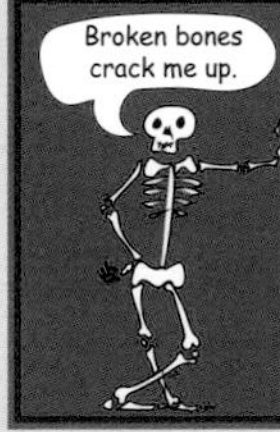

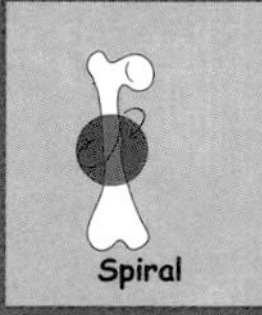

Spiral

Twisted break

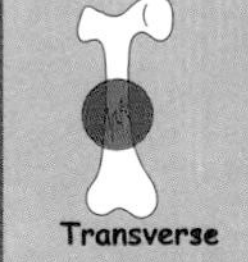

Transverse

Horizontal break

Greenstick

Partially bent, partially broken

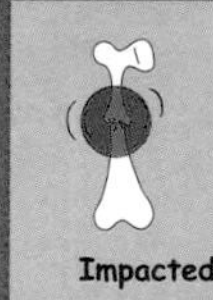

Impacted

Bone is wedged into the interior of the other

What You Need to Know

Types of Fractures

CLASSIFICATION OF FRACTURES

- **Complete**—break goes across the entire bone. The bone is actually divided into two sections.
- **Incomplete**—break does not go across the entire bone. The area may be splintered but not separated.
- **Open**—compound fracture that involves a break in the surface of the skin.
- **Closed**—simple fracture that does not break the surface of the skin.
- **Displaced**—bone fractures into two or more pieces and is misaligned.
- **Nondisplaced**—bone fractures but remains in alignment.

TYPES OF FRACTURES

- **Oblique**—simple fracture that may be complete or incomplete. The line of the fracture extends in an oblique direction across the bone.
  Cause—direct or indirect force across the bone with angulation
- **Occult**—fracture that is hidden and not immediately recognized. It is a simple fracture that is closed and most often not displaced.
  Cause—direct trauma force
- **Pathologic**—force that causes the break is significantly less than the force with other fractures. This type may spontaneously occur in patients with osteoporosis, tumors, or metastatic bone disease.
  Cause—bone disease, not an injury to the bone
- **Segmented**—fracture that results in several breaks. The bone is broken into at least two segmented pieces.
  Cause—direct or indirect force; moderate-to-severe force
- **Spiral**—fracture line that extends in a spiral pattern across the bone.
  Cause—direct or indirect twisting motion or twisting with distal part immobilized
- **Transverse**—complete fracture that has a horizontal break across the bone.
  Cause—direct or indirect force toward the bone
- **Greenstick**—Incomplete fracture that has a splintering of one side of the bone, rather than a break. This type is a very common fracture in children.
  Cause—direct or indirect force to an extremity

- **Impacted**—fracture with one or more bone fragments that are driven into each other. One end of the fracture may be wedged into the another fractured end.
  Cause—compression force or force distal to injured fragment

Important nursing implications | Serious/life-threatening implications
Most frequent side effects | Patient teaching

JOINT MOVEMENT

The function of the joints is to provide stability and movement to the body's form...

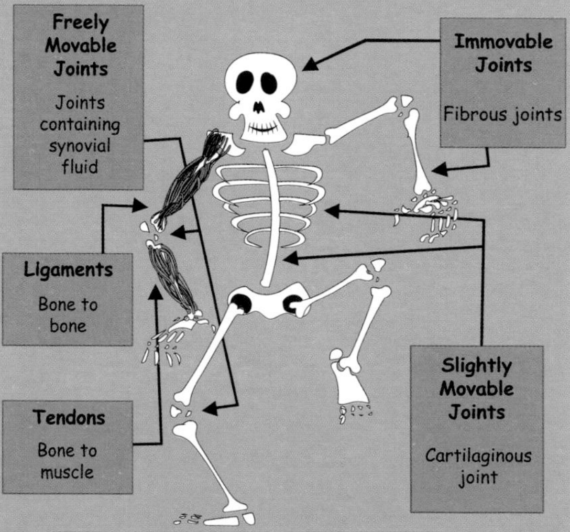

Freely Movable Joints

Joints containing synovial fluid

Immovable Joints

Fibrous joints

Ligaments

Bone to bone

Tendons

Bone to muscle

Slightly Movable Joints

Cartilaginous joint

A joint is classified by the degree of movement allowed by the connective tissues that hold the joint together. A joint allows movement by contraction, flexion, or relaxation.

What You Need to Know

Joint Movement

SIGNIFICANCE OF JOINT MOVEMENT

A joint occurs where two or more bones meet. Joints provide mobility and stability to the skeleton. Joints are classified by the amount of mobility the joint permits or the connecting tissues that hold the joint together.

TYPES OF JOINTS

- **Fibrous** (immovable)—degree of movement, if any, depends on the distance between the bones and the flexibility of the connective tissue. Examples of fibrous joints include those in the skull, as well as the paired bones of the lower arm and the lower leg.
- **Cartilaginous** (slightly movable)—allows some mobility. Movement is cushioned by a cartilage cushion and stabilizer. Examples of cartilaginous joints include those of the vertebrae and the symphysis pubis. Cartilage joints are also found at the ribs and the sternum.
- **Synovial** (fully movable)—the most common joint in the body has a fibrous joint capsule that covers the end of the articulating bones. The joint capsule has a rich blood and nerve supply and is capable of rapid healing. The joint cavity is an enclosed cavity filled with synovial fluid that enables the bones to move against each other. Synovial fluid cushions, lubricates, covers, and protects the ends of the articulating bones. Without the synovial fluid, the joint would rapidly deteriorate to immobility. Examples of synovial joints include the knees, elbows, fingers, and hips.

LIGAMENTS

- Ligaments have a poor blood supply and connect bones where they meet at the joints. Ligaments provide stability to a joint while allowing joint movement.
- *Sprain*—a tear of the ligament that surrounds the joint is classified according to the amount of damage that occurs to the ligaments and whether the joint has been made unstable.

TENDONS

- Tendons have a poor blood supply and attach the skeletal muscles to bones as an extension of the muscle.
- *Strain*—a tear in the tendon is the result of excessive stretching of the muscle and the facial sheath that involves the muscle and the tendons.

INFLAMMATORY JOINT DISEASE

Gouty Arthritis

Inflammatory response to deposits of uric acid crystals in a joint

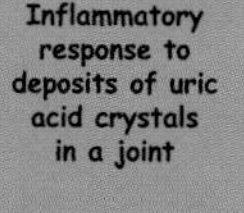

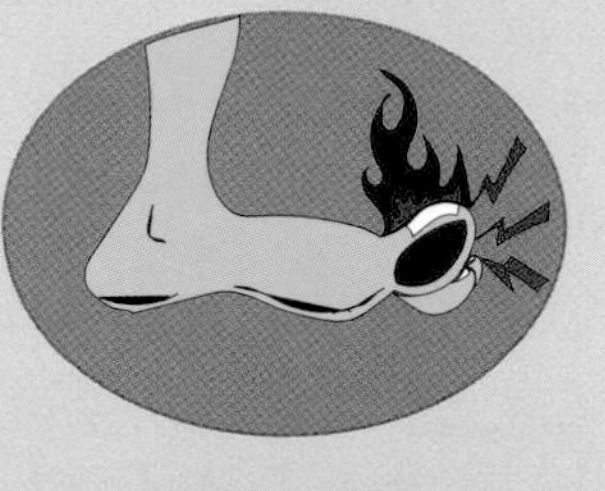

Rheumatoid Arthritis

Systemic autoimmune disease characterized by inflammation and damage to the synovial membrane and cartilage

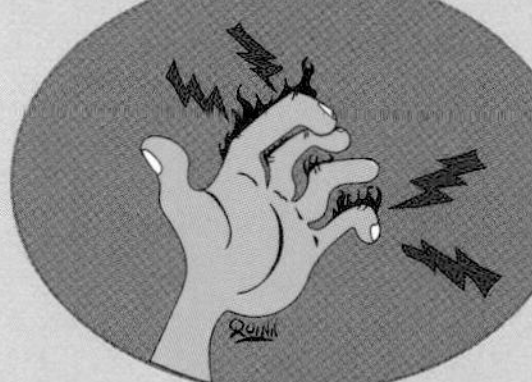

Ankylosing Spondylitis

Stiffening and fusion of spinal and sacroiliac joints, secondary to scar formation from inflammation

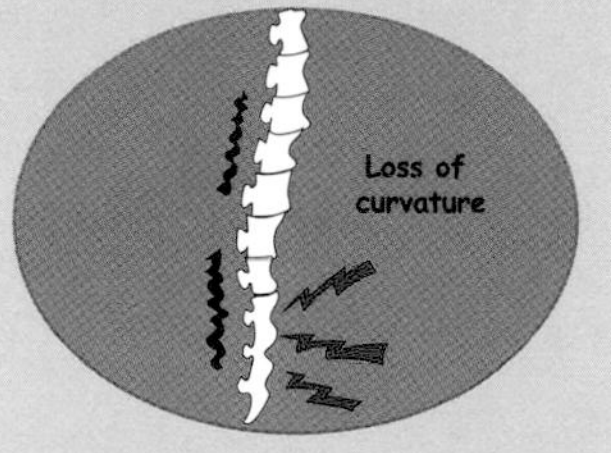

What You Need to Know

Inflammatory Joint Disease

GOUT

Gout is a systemic problem in which uric acid crystals are deposited in joints, which causes inflammation.

- Primary—is a problem of purine metabolism that causes excessive retention of uric acid and occurs more frequently in middle-aged to older males.
- Secondary—is related to another condition (e.g., excessive alcohol consumption, diuretic use, or chemotherapeutic medications).

Signs and Symptoms

- Increased levels of serum uric acid.
- May be precipitated by trauma, surgery, or systemic infection.
- Onset is frequently rapid with pain and swelling of the affected joint, most often the great toe. Patient is asymptomatic between attacks.

RHEUMATOID ARTHRITIS (RA)

- RA is an autoimmune disorder that most commonly affects the synovial joints.
- Autoantibodies (rheumatoid factors) are formed and cause progressive destructive inflammation in the joints.

Signs and Symptoms

- Rheumatoid factor is positive; C-reactive protein (CRP) levels increase.
- Pain and stiffness are more noticeable in the morning. Frequently affects the joints of the fingers and hands.
- Joints are swollen, painful, and warm to the touch. Involved joints are most often bilateral and symmetric. Morning stiffness may last from 1 to several hours.
- As the disease progresses, RA can affect all body systems.
- Single, swollen, inflamed joint may be an indication of infection.

ANKYLOSING SPONDYLITIS

- Chronic inflammatory disorder that primarily affects the vertebrae.
- Inflammation occurs in the synovial joint and adjacent tissue, forming granulation tissue and fibrous scars that fuse the tissue.

Signs and Symptoms

- Low back pain, stiffness, and limited movement are typical.

- Discomfort is frequently worse during the night and in the morning but decreases with mild activity.
- Postural deformities, decreased range of motion (ROM), kyphosis, lower-extremity weakness, and bladder dysfunction may occur.

Important nursing implications   Serious/life-threatening implications

Most frequent side effects   Patient teaching

JOINT DEGENERATION-OSTEOARTHRITIS

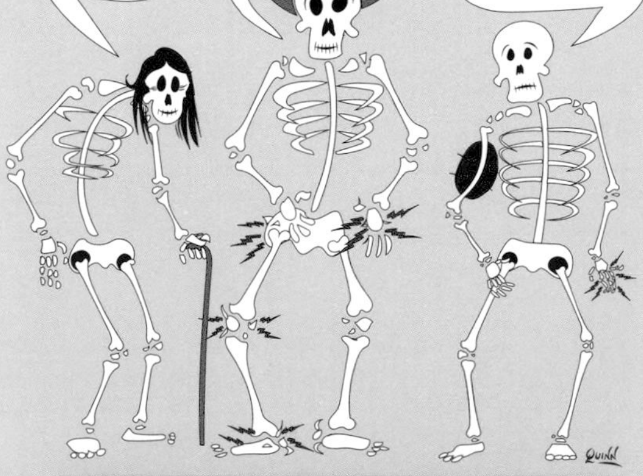

Idiopathic and secondary osteoarthritis have the same pathologic characteristics, but idiopathic osteoarthritis has an unknown origin. Idiopathic osteoarthitis is the most common type of noninflammatory joint disease.

What You Need to Know

Joint Degeneration—Osteoarthritis

SIGNIFICANCE OF OSTEOARTHRITIS

Osteoarthritis (OA) and *degenerative joint disease* (DJD) are common terms used to describe joint degeneration and are the most common forms of arthritis. OA is characterized by the progressive loss and deterioration of one or more joints. The weight-bearing joints such as the knees, hips, joints of the feet, and cervical and lumbar vertebrae are particularly affected.

- No specific cure is available.
- Continued changes in the cartilage lead to an erosion of the joint surface and structure.
- Inflammatory changes may occur within the joint, secondary to the irritation. Synovitis may also occur.
- As the condition progresses, cartilage is totally destroyed and the bony surfaces come in contact with one another, which results in increased pain and stiffness of the joint.

CAUSES

- Deterioration of cartilage and joints from normal aging process.
- Incidence increases in women and is linked to decreased estrogen.
- Majority of patients with OA are women over 50 years old.
- Trauma to a joint from excessive use or from abuse may also be a precipitating factor.
- Genetic factors appear to play a role in incidence.

SIGNS AND SYMPTOMS

- Joint pain is the predominant problem, and pain decreases with rest and increases with joint use. As the condition progresses, pain may occur with rest or during sleep.
- Crepitus, a grating sensation caused by the rubbing of the damaged joint, may be felt and heard.
- Joints are hypertrophied without any evidence of inflammation or heat.
- Heberden and Bouchard nodes are bony nodes that may appear on the hands and may be inflamed and painful.
- Early morning stiffness that generally resolves in 30 minutes.

CONGENITAL MUSCULOSKELETAL DEFECTS AND DEFORMITIES

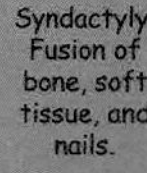

Syndactyly: Fusion of bone, soft tissue, and nails.

Polydactyly: one or more extra fingers.

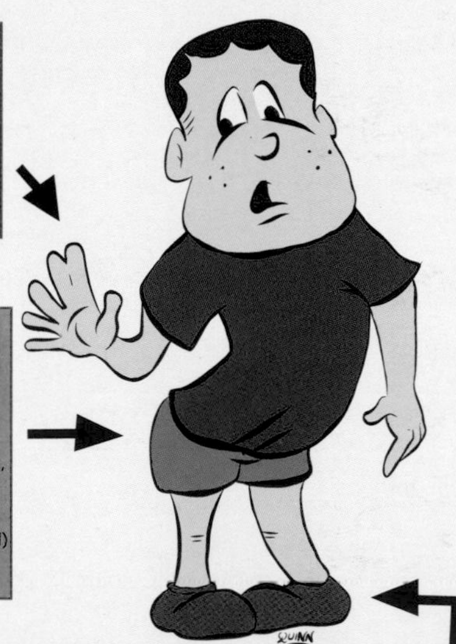

Developmental dysplasia of the hip: Abnormal development of the femur, the acetabulum, or both. Joint may be sublaxated (not well seated) or dislocated.

Talipes Equinovarus (clubfoot): Three Types

Positional: Easier to correct with casts	Idiopathic Congenital: Possible cast or surgical correction	Teratologic: Always requires surgical correction and muscle balancing

What You Need to Know

Congenital Musculoskeletal Defects and Deformities

SYNDACTYLY

- Is commonly referred to as *webbing* of the fingers or toes.
- Simple webbing involves only the soft tissue and is often corrected between 1 and 2 years of age.
- True syndactyly involves the fusion of the nails and bones. Surgery is usually required.

DEVELOPMENT DYSPLASIA OF THE HIP OR CONGENITAL HIP

- Condition involves the dislocation of the proximal femur or acetabulum (or both).
- Affected femur maintains contact with acetabulum but is not stable in the hip joint.
- Condition occurs in varying degrees of deformity and instability.

Signs and Symptoms

- Asymmetry of the gluteal folds
- Galeazzi sign—unequal leg length
- Limited abduction of affected hip
- Positive Ortolani sign or click as the femur moves in and out of the acetabulum

Treatment

Treatment is based on the severity and duration of the condition. The earlier the treatment, the better the prognosis. Abduction braces or devices, body casting, traction, or surgery may be recommended in children up to 1 year of age. Surgical correction becomes increasingly difficult after 4 years of age.

Congenital Clubfoot (Talipes Equinovarus)

Congenital clubfoot is a condition of the ankle and foot that involves bone deformity and malposition with contracture. The contracture is in adduction.

- Positional—occurs from intrauterine positioning and crowding.
- Idiopathic—cause is unknown; child has no other malformations.
- Teratologic—occurs with other congenital problems, such as spina bifida or myelomeningocele. This type is the most severe form and requires surgery.

TREATMENT

Treatment is based on the type of deformity. It may involve serial casting, bracing, or surgical intervention or any combination. Treatment usually begins shortly after birth.

Important nursing implications | Serious/life-threatening implications

Most frequent side effects | Patient teaching

AGING AND MUSCULOSKELETAL SYSTEM FUNCTION

Pregnancy, menopause, and low levels of calcium cause deformity, pain, stiffness, and increased fractures.

Decreased testosterone occurs later in life and increases the process of bone loss.

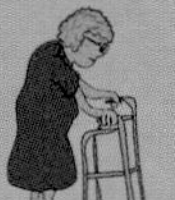

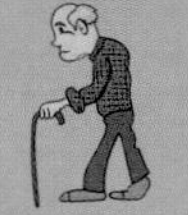

Aging Bones

Decreased space between intervertebral disks can cause a decrease in height.

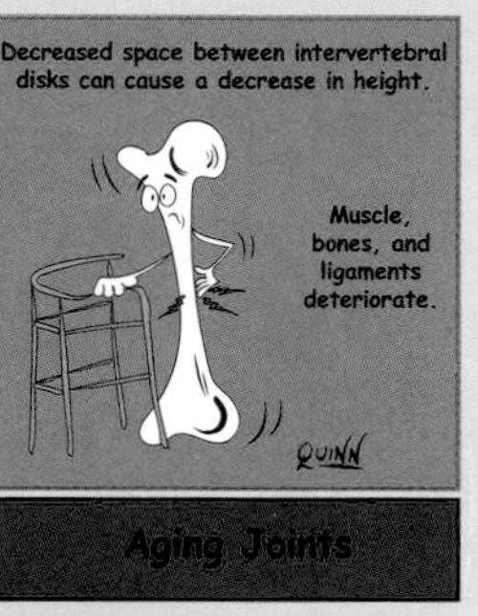

Muscle, bones, and ligaments deteriorate.

Aging Joints

Muscle fibers begin to break down.

Changes in vascular, endocrine, and nervous systems lead to poor muscle quality.

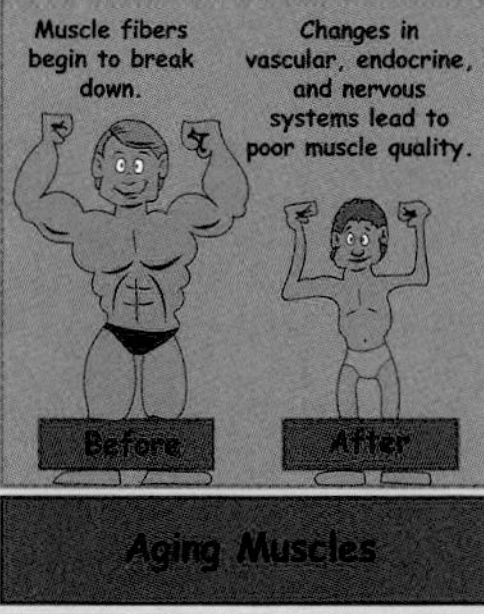

Aging Muscles

Muscle bulk and strength slowly decline with aging.
Bone loss can be related to smoking, increased alcohol use, physical inactivity, and low calcium, magnesium, and vitamin D.

What You Need to Know

Aging and Musculoskeletal System Function

AGING BONES

- Bones become stiff, weak, and brittle with aging.
- Women experience more problems with decreased bone density as a result of the effects of increased bone loss during pregnancy and menopause.
- Bone loss can be extensive enough (osteoporosis) to cause pathologic fractures, deformity (kyphosis), and vertebral compression fractures.
- Bone loss in males is slower than in females and is related to testosterone levels, physical activity, and heredity.
- Bone loss may also be attributed to smoking, calcium, magnesium, and vitamin D deficiency. Alcohol, drug use, and some prescription medications may also contribute to bone loss.

AGING JOINTS

- Cartilage in the joints develops layers with deep fissures (fibrillation).
- Cartilage becomes thin and absent in areas, leaving the bones unprotected.
- OA is a degenerative joint disease associated with aging.
- Vertebral joints in the cervical area and in the lower lumbar area become compressed, causing a decrease in height.

AGING MUSCLES

- Healthy muscles depend not only on healthy muscle fiber but also on adequate functioning of the endocrine, nervous, and vascular systems.
- Decreased metabolic rate occurs with aging.
- Muscle strength and bulk decline slowly.
- Age-related loss of muscle tissue and strength is called *sarcopenia.*
- Aging causes the muscles to lose strength and bulk; decreased strength is evident in the seventh decade of life; however, muscles can be trainable even into advanced age.
- Strength training can increase muscle mass and strength as well as slow the rate of bone loss.
- Balance and coordination exercises can reduce the risk of falls.
- Stretching helps maintain joint flexibility.

ALTERATIONS IN OCULAR MOVEMENTS

VISUAL DYSFUNCTION

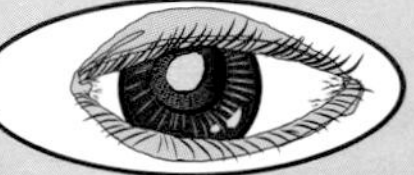

My eyes are bouncing all over the page.

Involuntary, unilateral or bilateral, or rhythmic eye movement may occur when at rest or with use.

Nystagmus

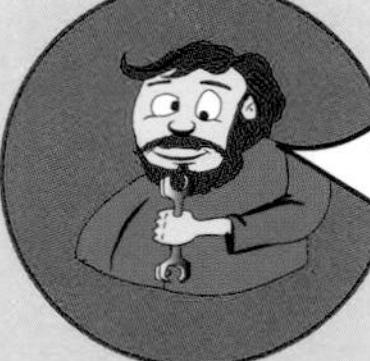

I see two of everything.

Deviation of one eye occurs when focusing on an object. Causes diplopia.

Strabismus

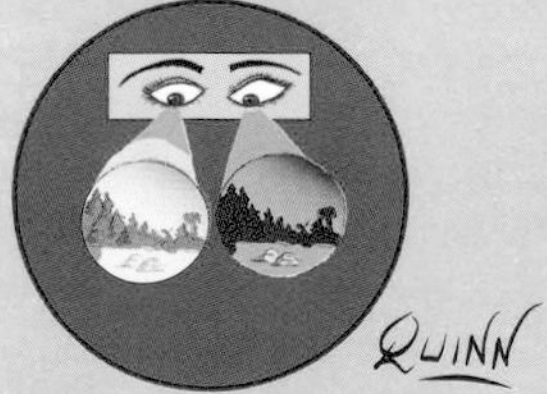

Without treatment, strabismus could lead to a reduction in vision of the affected eye, known as amblyopia.

Amblyopia

What You Need to Know

Alterations in Ocular Movements—Visual Dysfunction

SIGNIFICANCE OF OCULAR MOVEMENTS

Abnormal ocular movements occur as a result of problems with the cranial nerves (CNs) that control the ocular muscles.

- **Oculomotor (CN III)**—controls motor fibers to the muscles that move the eyeball. These muscles affect the ability of the eye to track movement, as well as pupil size and reflex.
- **Trochlear (CN IV)**—controls motor fibers for the external eye muscle. These muscles control the ability of the eye to follow moving objects.
- **Abducens (CN VI)**—controls motor fibers to the lateral rectus muscle and is evaluated according to the ability of each eye to move laterally.

STRABISMUS

- One eye deviates from the point of fixation.
- If the problem is constant, then the weak eye becomes "lazy," and the brain will eventually suppress the image from that eye. If the problem is not corrected, **amblyopia** or blindness in the eye from disuse can result.
- *Common tests*—cover test and corneal light reflex are important diagnostic tools.

NYSTAGMUS

- Abnormal involuntary rhythmic repetitive movement of the eye either horizontal, vertical, or rotary.
- Problem may be caused by the movement of the endolymph fluid in the inner ear. Nystagmus occurs in patients with labyrinthitis, lesions of the central nervous system (CNS), and drug toxicity.
- *Common test*—ask the patient to look straight ahead and follow the examiner's finger to an extreme lateral gaze. Quick jerking movements of the eye are indicative of nystagmus.

PARALYSIS

- Occurs with paralysis of the extraocular muscles.
- Problems occur as a result of unopposed muscle activity.
- Diseases such as diabetes mellitus, multiple sclerosis, and myasthenia gravis may affect specific extraocular muscles.

- *Common test*—is nonspecific. Patient is unable to move the eye or focus on an object.

Important nursing implications	Serious/life-threatening implications
Most frequent side effects	Patient teaching

ALTERATIONS IN VISUAL ACUITY

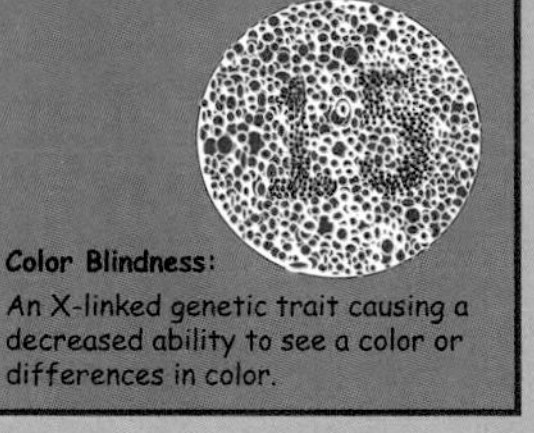

Color Blindness:
An X-linked genetic trait causing a decreased ability to see a color or differences in color.

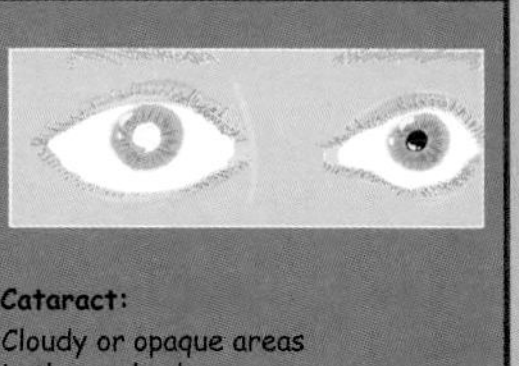

Cataract:
Cloudy or opaque areas in the ocular lens.

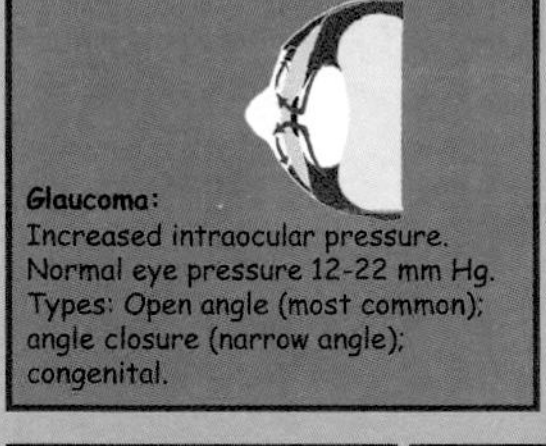

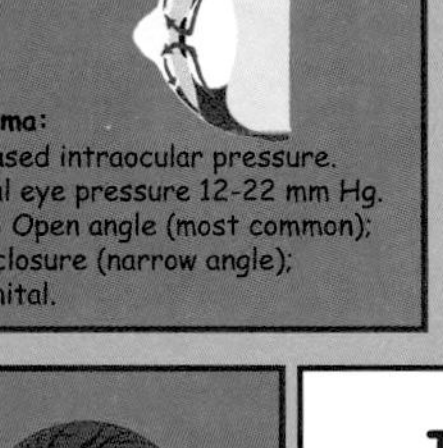

Glaucoma:
Increased intraocular pressure.
Normal eye pressure 12-22 mm Hg.
Types: Open angle (most common); angle closure (narrow angle); congenital.

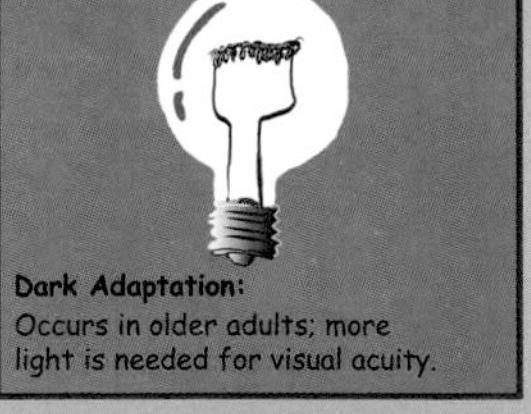

Dark Adaptation:
Occurs in older adults; more light is needed for visual acuity.

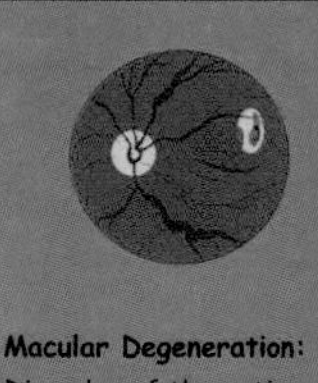

Macular Degeneration:
Disorder of the retina causing loss of central vision in people over age 60 years.

I
CAN
NOT
SEEA
THING

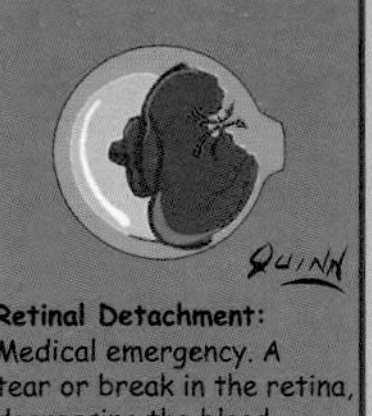

Retinal Detachment:
Medical emergency. A tear or break in the retina, decreasing the blood supply, oxygen, and nourishment to the area.

What You Need to Know

Alterations in Visual Acuity

CATARACTS

- Opacity of the ocular lens, decreased acuity, and blurred vision are indicative of cataracts.
- Incidence increases with age, and cataracts can be surgically removed and a prosthetic lens placed.

PAPILLEDEMA

- Inflammation and edema of the optic nerve develops where the nerve enters the eyeball.
- Optic disk may become raised above the level of the retina.
- Problem occurs with increased intracranial pressure (ICP), neuritis, and changes in retinal blood vessels.

RETINAL DETACHMENT

- Fluid or a retinal tear separates the retina from the choroid and decreases the blood supply to the retina.
- May occur as a retinal break or hole in the retina. If left untreated, then retinal detachment frequently leads to blindness in the affected eye.

MACULAR DEGENERATION

- Loss of central vision occurring generally in individuals over age 60.
- Loss of the outer retina occurs along with pigment of the macula.
- Scar tissue and bleeding develop, causing retinal detachment.
- Older patients may experience blurred vision, difficulty reading, and poor night vision.

DARK ADAPTATION

- Patient requires more light to see due to loss of visual acuity.
- Individual at 80 years old requires twice as much light as a 20 year old.

GLAUCOMA

- Increased intraocular pressure is sustained. Normal pressure is 12–22 mm Hg.
- Primary open-angle glaucoma is the most common form and develops slowly.

- Peripheral vision is severely compromised. Repair of damaged vision is not possible.

COLOR BLINDNESS

- X-linked genetic trait.
- Decreased ability to distinguish certain colors, especially shades of green and red.

Important nursing implications
Serious/life-threatening implications
Most frequent side effects
Patient teaching

ALTERATIONS IN REFRACTION

MYOPIA
I can see near things but not distant things.

HYPEROPIA
I can see far things but not close things.
QUINN

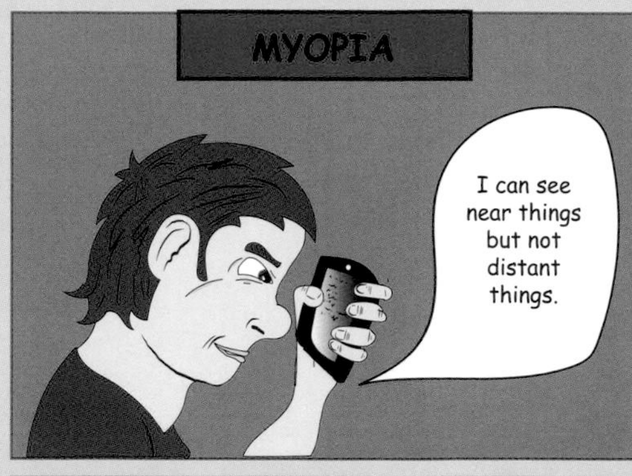

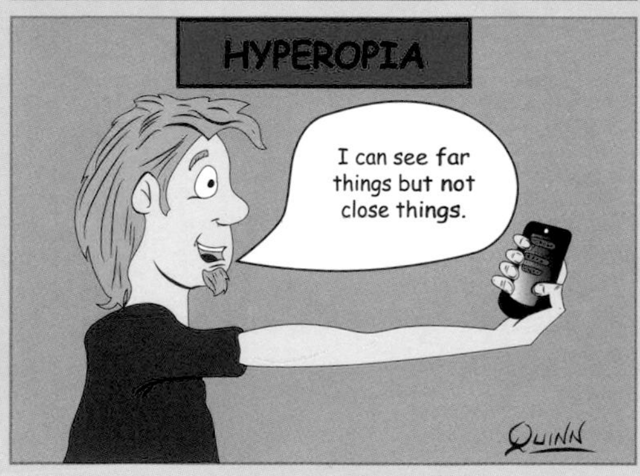

What You Need to Know

Alterations in Refraction

SIGNIFICANCE OF REFRACTION

Refraction is the ability of the eye to focus light rays through the lens to an image on the retina. When the shape of the eye prevents light rays from focusing on the retina, it is referred to as a *refraction error*. Refraction errors are the most common of visual problems and are corrected by some type of alteration to the lens. Glasses, contact lens, or surgical correction is available to correct refractive errors.

SIGNS, SYMPTOMS, AND MANAGEMENT

- Blurred vision is the primary symptom.
- Treatment options include corrective lenses (glasses, contacts) or surgery (LASIK).

TYPES OF REFRACTIVE ERRORS

Myopia (Nearsightedness)

- An image in the distance becomes focused in front of the retina. The individual experiences blurred distant vision and clear close vision and frequently squints to try to improve vision.
- Problem may also be caused by a swelling of the lens in patients with diabetes mellitus. This problem is transient and resolves with the correction of blood glucose levels.
- Cause may be from too long of eyeball axis, or the refractive power of the eye is too strong.

Hyperopia (Farsightedness)

- Most common refractive error.
- An image in the distance becomes focused behind the retina. The individual can see distant objects clearly, but near objects are blurred (e.g., reading).
- Cause may be from too short of eyeball axis, or the refractive power of the eye is too weak.

Presbyopia

- Is different from nearsightedness and farsightedness.
- Age-related process that is believed to stem from a gradual loss of flexibility in the natural lens of the eye.
- Inability to focus on near objects because of insufficient accommodation ability.

NURSING IMPLICATIONS

- Encourage all patients, especially those with diabetes, to have annual eye examinations.

Important nursing implications

Serious/life-threatening implications

Most frequent side effects

Patient teaching

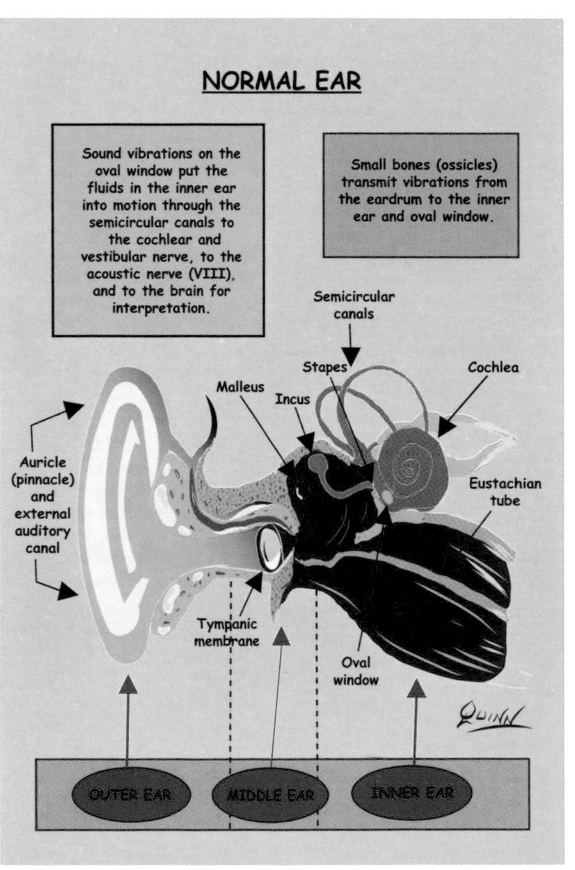
NORMAL EAR
Sound vibrations on the oval window put the fluids in the inner ear into motion through the semicircular canals to the cochlear and vestibular nerve, to the acoustic nerve (VIII), and to the brain for interpretation.
Small bones (ossicles) transmit vibrations from the eardrum to the inner ear and oval window.
Semicircular canals
Stapes
Cochlea
Malleus
Incus
Auricle (pinnacle) and external auditory canal
Eustachian tube
Tympanic membrane
Oval window
QUINN
OUTER EAR
MIDDLE EAR
INNER EAR

What You Need to Know

Normal Ear

OUTER OR EXTERNAL EAR

- The outer or external ear is responsible for the collection of sound waves and funnelling these waves through the ear canal to the tympanic membrane.
- The tympanic membrane separates the outer ear from the middle ear.

MIDDLE EAR

- The middle ear consists of three small auditory ossicle bones: (1) malleus, (2) incus, and (3) stapes. This ossicular chain is responsible for the movement of the sound waves into the inner ear. A direct connection between the middle ear and the eustachian tube allows for the equalization of atmospheric pressure.
- The external and middle ear amplify sound waves from the outside. These areas are primarily responsible for hearing defects that are classified as *conductive hearing loss.*
- The middle ear is also the location of *otitis media,* the most common ear infection.

INNER EAR

- The inner ear begins where the stapes *interface*s with the oval window. The inner ear contains the organs for hearing and for balance.
- The inner ear has a series of bony labyrinths—the cochlea, vestibule, and semicircular canals.
- The receptor organ for hearing is the cochlea. It contains tiny hairlike cells that form the organ of Corti, which produces nerve impulses in response to sound vibrations.
- Once the sound stimulates the bony labyrinth, the sound is transmitted to the cochlea, where it is picked up by the vestibulocochlear nerve (CN VIII) and then to the auditory cortex of the temporal lobe of the brain for interpretation.
- Problems with the nerve pathway in the inner ear are referred to as *sensorineural hearing loss.*
- The semicircular canals of the inner ear are also responsible for equilibrium. The membranous labyrinth is filled with a thick fluid or gel called the endolymphatic fluid. Receptors are located here and are directly responsible for an individual's sense of balance.

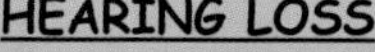

HEARING LOSS

Outer Ear Problems:
- Wax impaction
- Foreign bodies
- Otitis external

Middle Ear Problems:
- Otitis media
- Serous otitis
- Otosclerosis

Inner Ear Problems:
- Meniere disease
- Noise exposure
- Ototoxicity

I can't hear you clearly.

QUINN

Conductive Hearing Loss:
Occurs in the outer and middle ear. Sound is impaired from being conducted to the inner ear.

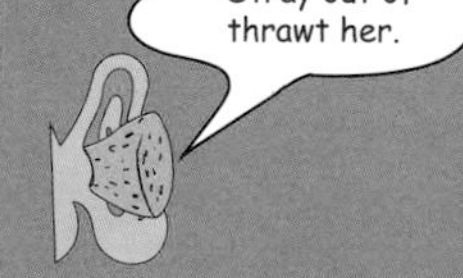

Sensorineural Hearing Loss:
Occurs in the inner ear. Sound may be heard but cannot be correctly interpreted.

Stay out of the water.

What You Need to Know

Hearing Loss

OUTER EAR

- Problems that occur in the outer ear interfere with the transmission of sound into the middle ear.
- Problems are most often characterized by something that blocks the movement of the sound waves, which may be a foreign object or an infection with swelling, drainage, and pain.

MIDDLE EAR

- Otitis media is the most common infection and occurs most often in children under 3 years of age. The eustachian tube is shorter and more open in young children.
- Age-related changes also occur in the middle ear. Otosclerosis occurs in the auditory ossicles and the transmission of sound is impaired, which may be referred to as *conductive hearing loss.* The individual with conductive hearing loss will benefit from a hearing aid.

INNER EAR

- Cochlea and the organ of Corti are sensitive to aging changes.
- *Presbycusis* is the inability to hear high-frequency sounds.
- The inability to determine the location of sound may be a result of aging and may occur in one ear or bilaterally. This problem is referred to as *sensorineural hearing loss* and involves nerves and the interpretation of the sounds. The individual experiences hearing loss, difficulty interpreting speech, and tinnitus. The hearing loss may be gradual or sudden.
- Medications, especially the aminoglycoside family of antibiotics, affect hearing in the inner ear. The individual with a sensorineural hearing loss does not benefit from a hearing aid.
- **Meniere disease** is characterized by symptoms that reflect problems with the balance mechanism in the inner ear. The patient with Meniere disease will experience imbalance, vertigo, and tinnitus. It is frequently episodic and may be bilateral.
- The older person with hearing difficulties may also experience a mixed—both conductive and sensorineural—hearing loss.

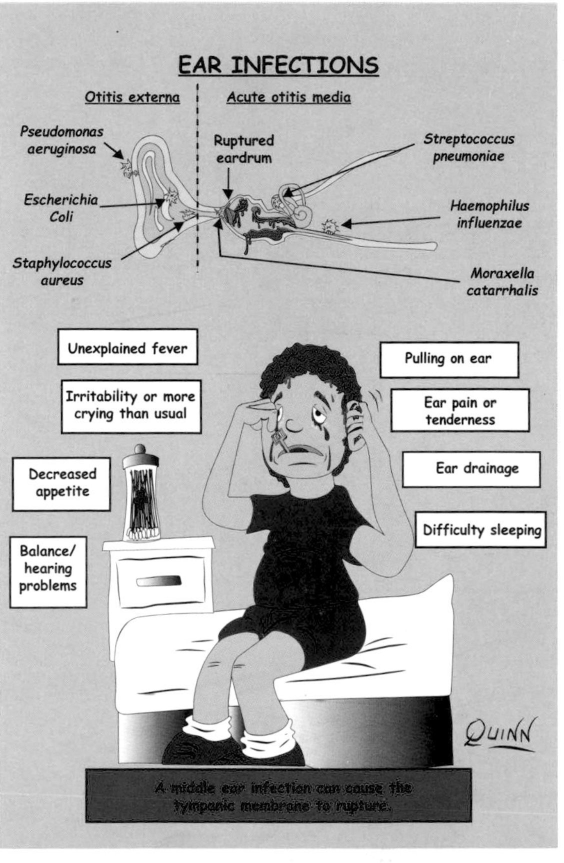
EAR INFECTIONS
Otitis externa
Acute otitis media
Pseudomonas aeruginosa
Escherichia Coli
Staphylococcus aureus
Ruptured eardrum
Streptococcus pneumoniae
Haemophilus influenzae
Moraxella catarrhalis
Unexplained fever
Irritability or more crying than usual
Decreased appetite
Balance/ hearing problems
Pulling on ear
Ear pain or tenderness
Ear drainage
Difficulty sleeping
QUINN
A middle ear infection can cause the tympanic membrane to rupture.

What You Need to Know

Ear Infections

OTITIS EXTERNA

- Infection of the outer ear—inflammation occurs when water is trapped in the external canal by bathing or swimming. Normally, wax protects the ear canal and is secreted from the sebaceous glands.
- May also be the result of a foreign body or trauma. *Pseudomonas aeruginosa* and *Staphylococcus aureus* are the most common pathogens.

Signs and Symptoms

- Pain and conductive hearing loss may be present.
- As the problem progresses, the pain becomes more intense.
- Ear is more sensitive to touch, and drainage may occur from the ear canal.

ACUTE OTITIS MEDIA

- Infection in the middle ear—one of the most common problems in children aged 3 years and younger. The eustachian tube is short, wide, and straight in infants and children. The mechanical obstruction of the eustachian tube and the accumulation of secretions in the middle ear precipitate the problem.
- Is frequently associated with upper respiratory conditions, bottle-fed infants, and infants exposed to passive smoke. Eardrum perforation is a common complication.
- Most often the eardrum will heal, but multiple perforations may necessitate surgical intervention and result in hearing loss.

Sign and Symptoms

- Pain occurs as a result of pressure on surrounding tissue.
- Purulent fluid accumulates in the middle ear.
- Infants may pull at their ears, be very irritable, anorexic, and have difficulty sucking.
- Fever is frequently high, and cervical lymph glands are enlarged.
- Diagnosis is based on clinical manifestations.

Important nursing implications | Serious/life-threatening implications

Most frequent side effects | Patient teaching

PROBLEMS IN THE CNS

Altered Level of Consciousness:

Caused by change or an increase in the intracranial pressure.

Hey, can you hear me? Wake up.... wiggle your toes!

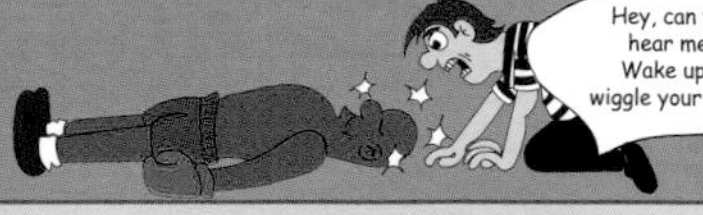

Pain Response:

Sensations move along neuropathic ways to bring information to the brain.

Afferent neurons sends a signal to the brain...."Hot!"
Efferent neurons sends a signal from the brain to your hand..."Move your hand!"

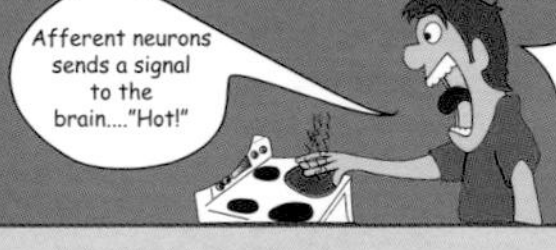

Altered Gaits:

Central nervous system problems can be seen in gait changes.

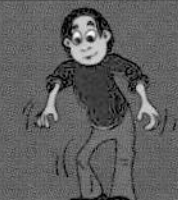

- Spastic gait
- Scissors gait
- Cerebellar gait
- Basal ganglion gait
- Senile gait

Nausea and Vomiting:

The brainstem is connected to the central nervous system; nausea and vomiting can occur from stimulation of this area.

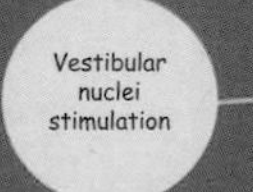

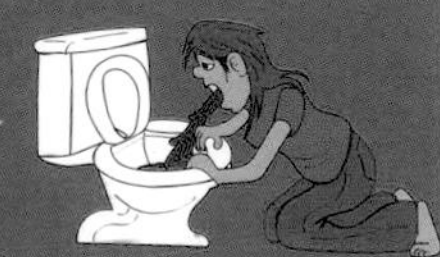

Muscle Tone:

- Hypotonia—Decreased muscle tone. Weak or flaccid movements from interruption of nerve impulses.
- Hypertonia—Muscles are stiff and difficult to move from constant muscle stimulation.
- Rigidity—Increased muscle tone. Stiffness or inflexible muscles from increased nerve impulses.
- Dystonia—Involuntary muscle contractions that cause slow repetitive movements.

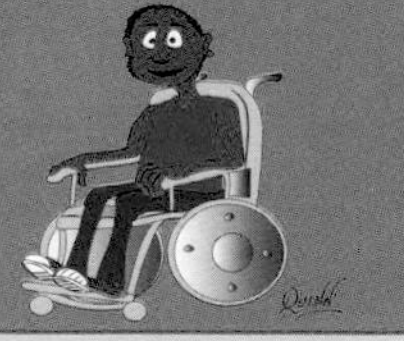

What You Need to Know

Nervous System

ALTERED LEVEL OF CONSCIOUSNESS

Consciousness has two distinct components: (1) arousal and (2) awareness.

- Arousal—attentional system; state of awakeness is mediated by the reticular-activating system. Coma is the primary symptom of an arousable state.
- Awareness—all cognitive functions embody awareness of self, environment, and affective states. Common symptoms include sensory inattentiveness (neglect) and memory deficits.

NAUSEA AND VOMITING

- Stimulation of the vestibular nuclei in the brainstem leads to nausea and vomiting.
- Projectile vomiting is often associated with brainstem lesions.

ALTERED GAITS

Complex motor movements, such as disorders of posture (stance) and gait, occur with central nervous system (CNS) problems.

- Posture (stance)—dystonic (choreoathetoid movements), decerebrate (extensor posturing), and decorticate (flexor posturing)
- Gait disorders—spastic (type of upper motor neuron associated with unilateral injury), scissors (associated with bilateral injury and spasticity with damage to pyramidal system), cerebellar (ataxic, wide-based gait; staggering noted), and basal ganglion and senile gait (broad-based, small steps with diminished arm swing)

PAIN RESPONSE

- Alteration in interpretation of pain stimuli along the neuropathic pathway as a result of intracranial pressure (ICP), traumatic injury, or brain tumor can lead to a pain response.

MUSCLE TONE

- Hypotonia—extremities are floppy; flaccidity is associated with limp, atrophied muscles, and paralysis.
- Hypertonia—spasticity, dystonia (sustained involuntary twisting movement), and rigidity (lead-pipe, cogwheel) are noted.

Important nursing implications	Serious/life-threatening implications
Most frequent side effects	Patient teaching

PAIN

Somatic Pain

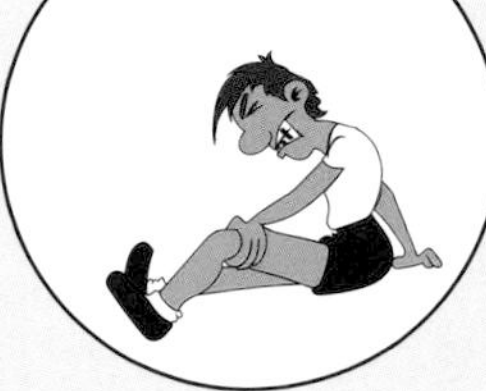

Affects skin, muscles, ligaments, tendons, and joints. Localized, intense pain.

Visceral Pain

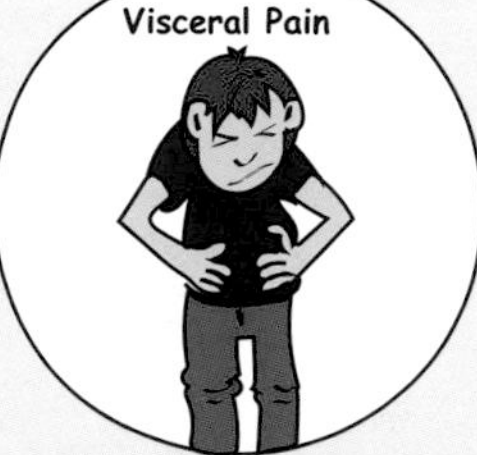

Affects the internal organs. Poorly localized, dull, aching, and vague pain.

Acute Pain

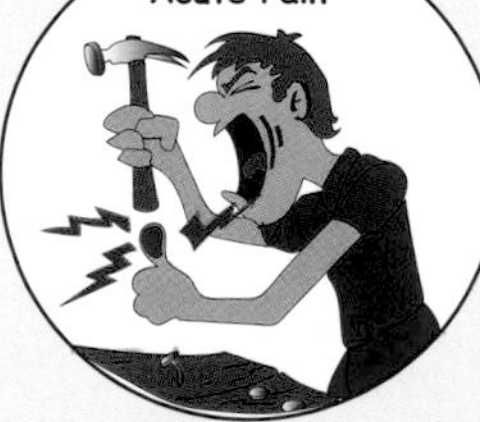

A normal protective mechanism that is transient, lasting from seconds to days and up to 3 months. Begins suddenly and is sharp in quality. May cause increased heart rate, hypertension, diaphoresis, and dilated pupils.

Chronic Pain

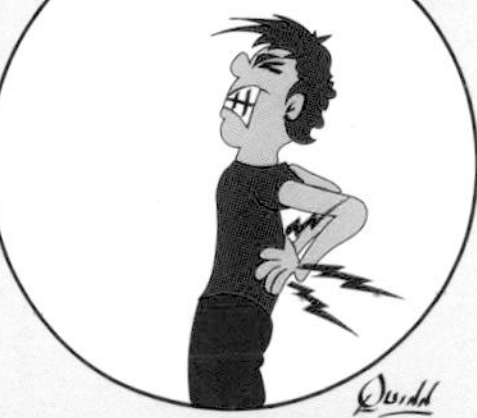

Lasts more than 6 months and can be ongoing (low back pain) or intermittent (migraine headaches). May cause muscle tension, lack of energy, change in appetite, depression, or anxiety. Can continue after injury or illness is gone.

What You Need to Know

Pain

SIGNIFICANCE OF PAIN

Pain is an unpleasant personal experience and defined as whatever the individual experiencing the pain says it is. An action potential is generated and converts the pain stimulus to an impulse, sending it to the spinal cord.

ANATOMY OF PAIN

- Afferent pathways carry the pain signal to the spinal cord and then to the brain.
- CNS interprets the pain signal—fight or flight response is activated.
- Perception is the conscious awareness of the pain.
- Efferent pathways carry signals away from the brain (CNS).

CLASSIFICATION OF PAIN

Pain can be classified according to its underlying pathologic classification.

- **Nociceptive pain**—(normal processing of noxious stimuli) that may occur due to a broken bone, surgical incision, or cardiac ischemia
  - The cause of nociceptive pain is from damage to somatic or visceral tissue.
  - Somatic pain: Aching or throbbing pain that is well localized and generally intense. Arises from bone, joint, muscle, tendons, ligaments, skin, or connective tissue.
  - Visceral pain: Dull, aching, poorly localized, vague pain that may result from stimuli such as tumor involvement or obstruction. Arises from internal organs such as the intestines and bladder.
- **Neuropathic pain**—(abnormal pain processing) that may be seen with phantom limb pain or diabetic neuropathies
  - Damage to nerve cells or changes in spinal cord processing causes neuropathic pain.
  - Described as burning, shooting, or stabbing; may also be referred pain.

ACUTE OR CHRONIC CLASSIFICATION

Acute

- Onset is sudden; heart rate, respiratory rate, and blood pressure increase with acute pain.
- Pain is mild to severe, generally lasts less than 3 months, and decreases over time.
- Behavior includes anxiety, confusion, and agitation.

Chronic

- Pain does not go away and lasts for 6 months or more. Waxing and waning are characteristic of chronic pain.
- Cause of pain may not be known.
- Behavior includes withdrawal, decreased physical movement, and fatigue.

Important nursing implications

Serious/life-threatening implications

Most frequent side effects

Patient teaching

BLOOD-BRAIN BARRIER

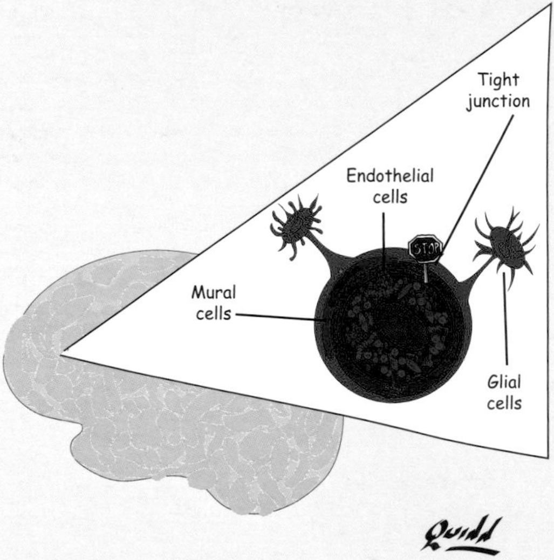

Tight junction

Endothelial cells

Mural cells

Glial cells

STOP!

Quidd

The blood brain barrier protects the brain from bacteria, viruses, and toxins. It selectively inhibits substances in the blood from entering the interstitial spaces of the brain or cerebral spinal fluid. Endothelial cells, mural cells, glial cells, and tight junctions work together to form the barrier.

What You Need to Know

Blood–Brain Barrier

SIGNIFICANCE OF THE BLOOD–BRAIN BARRIER

The *blood–brain barrier* (BBB) is a semipermeable barrier between blood capillaries and brain tissue. The *choroid plexus* and *arachnoid membrane*, made of endothelial cells, mural cells, glial cells, and tight junctions, act together as barriers between the blood and cerebrospinal fluid (CSF) creating the BBB. The BBB blocks all molecules except those that cross cell membranes by means of lipid solubility (e.g., oxygen, carbon dioxide, anesthetics, ethanol) and those that are allowed in by specific transport systems (e.g., sugars, some amino acids).

Many medications, as well as albumin and other hydrophilic substances, are unable to pass the barrier. This barrier can have implications when treating problems with brain tissue.

FUNCTIONS OF THE BLOOD–BRAIN BARRIER

- Protects the brain from *foreign substances* in the blood that may injure the brain.
- Protects the brain from hormones and neurotransmitters secreted by other organs of the body.
- Maintains a constant biochemical environment for the brain.

WHAT CAN INCREASE THE PERMEABILITY OF OR BREAK DOWN THE BLOOD–BRAIN BARRIER?

- Hypertension
- Dilutional hypernatremia
- High doses of some anesthetics
- Vasodilation
- Hypercapnia

Important nursing implications | Serious/life-threatening implications

Most frequent side effects | Patient teaching

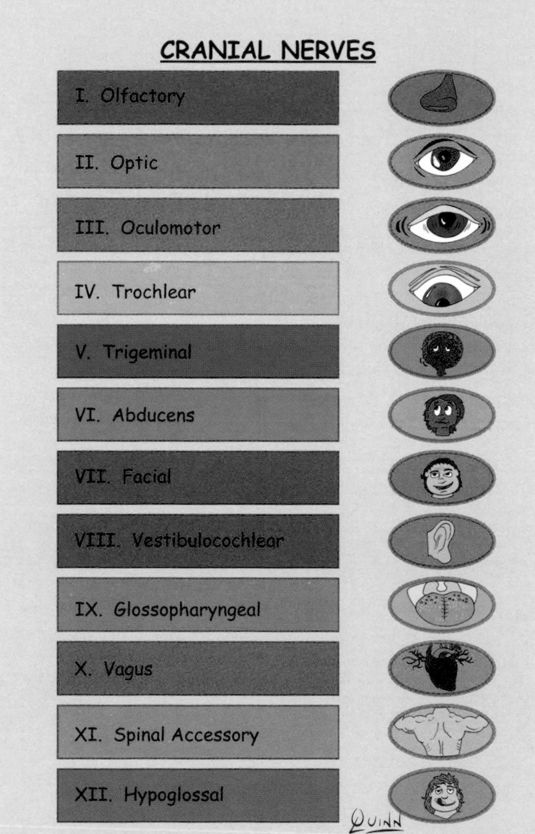
CRANIAL NERVES
I. Olfactory
II. Optic
III. Oculomotor
IV. Trochlear
V. Trigeminal
VI. Abducens
VII. Facial
VIII. Vestibulocochlear
IX. Glossopharyngeal
X. Vagus
XI. Spinal Accessory
XII. Hypoglossal
QUINN

What You Need to Know

Cranial Nerves

SIGNIFICANCE OF CRANIAL NERVES

There are 12 pairs of cranial nerves composed of cell bodies with fibers that exit the cranial cavity. Unlike the spinal nerves, they have both motor and sensory fibers. The cranial nerves can have only motor or sensory nerves or both.

Mnemonic to Remember Names of the Cranial Nerves

- **O**n **O**ld **O**lympus' **T**iny **T**op **A** **F**inn **A**nd **G**erman **V**iewed **S**ome **H**ops
- The **BOLDED** letters stand for **O**lfactory, **O**ptic, **O**culomotor, **T**rochlear, **T**rigeminal, **A**bducens, **F**acial, **A**uditory, **G**lossopharyngeal, **V**agus, **A**ccessory, and **H**ypoglossal.

Mnemonic to Remember Whether Nerve Is Sensory, Motor, or Both

- Some Say **M**arry **M**oney, **B**ut **M**y **B**rother Says **B**ad **B**usiness **M**arrying **M**oney

Cranial Nerve	Sensory or Motor	Major Functions
I Olfactory	Sensory	Smell
II Optic	Sensory	Vision
III Oculomotor	Motor	Eye movement laterally, horizontally, inward; eyelid elevation; eye focus; pupil constriction; accommodation
IV Trochlear	Motor	Innervates superior oblique muscle
V Trigeminal	Both	Turns eye downward and laterally Biting, chewing, and swallowing Touch, pain, and temperature sensation from face and scalp
VI Abducens	Motor	Moves eye laterally
VII Facial	Both	Controls most facial expressions
VIII Vestibulocochlear (acoustic)	Sensory	Secretion of tears and saliva Taste Hearing
IX Glossopharyngeal	Both	Sense of equilibrium Taste

Cranial Nerve	Sensory or Motor	Major Functions
X Vagus	Both	Gag reflex Senses carotid blood pressure Senses aortic blood pressure
XI Spinal accessory	Motor	Slows HR Stimulates digestive organs Controls trapezius and sternocleidomastoid muscles
XII Hypoglossal	Motor	Controls swallowing movements Controls tongue movements

Important nursing implications

Serious/life-threatening implications

Most frequent side effects

Patient teaching

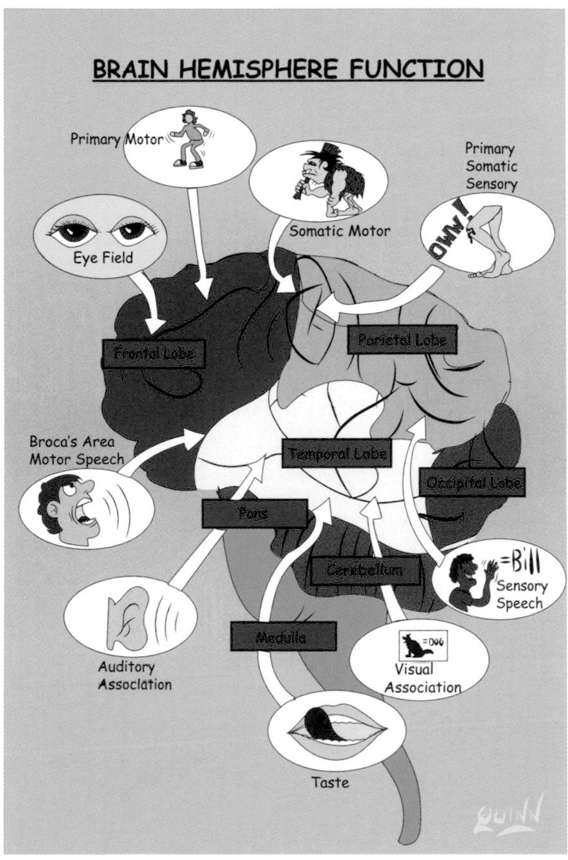
BRAIN HEMISPHERE FUNCTION
Primary Motor
Somatic Motor
Primary Somatic Sensory
OWW!
Eye Field
Frontal Lobe
Parietal Lobe
Broca's Area Motor Speech
Temporal Lobe
Occipital Lobe
Pons
Cerebellum
=Bill
Sensory Speech
Medulla
=DOG
Auditory Association
Visual Association
Taste
QUINN

What You Need to Know

Brain Hemisphere Function

SIGNIFICANCE OF BRAIN HEMISPHERE FUNCTION

The two hemispheres of the brain serve different functions and process information differently.

HEMISPHERES

Left Hemisphere

- Focuses on detail and is sequential, logical, and analytical.
- Performs better at tasks that entail discrete steps.
- Decodes the sequence and structure of language.

Right Hemisphere

- Holistically processes information and is associated with imagination and spatial perception.
- Performs better at understanding humor, emotion, and metaphor.

LOBES

Frontal

- Cognition and memory
  - Prefrontal area—has the ability to concentrate and conducts elaboration of thought.
  - Is the *gatekeeper* for judgment, decision-making, and inhibition.
  - Personality and emotional traits reside here.
- Voluntary Movement
  - Motor cortex (Brodmann area)—controls voluntary motor activity.
  - Broca's area—language—controls motor speech.

Parietal

- Processes sensory input, sensory discrimination, and body orientation.
- Identification of objects and understand spatial relationships.
- Wernicke's area—understand spoken language.

Occipital

- Controls primary visual reception area and visual association.

Temporal

- Short-term memory—integrates memories with sensations of taste, sound, sight, and touch. Controls auditory receptive area and association areas.

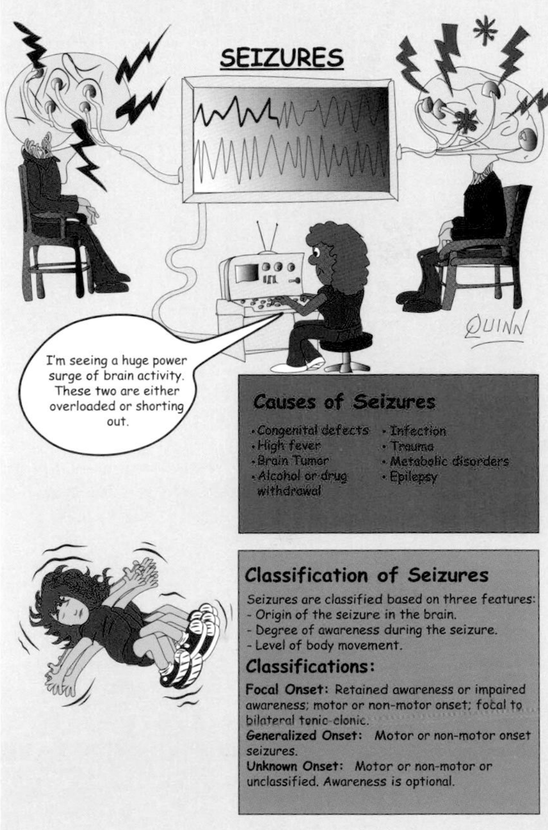
SEIZURES
QUINN
I'm seeing a huge power surge of brain activity. These two are either overloaded or shorting out.
Causes of Seizures
• Congenital defects
• High fever
• Brain Tumor
• Alcohol or drug withdrawal
• Infection
• Trauma
• Metabolic disorders
• Epilepsy
Classification of Seizures
Seizures are classified based on three features:
- Origin of the seizure in the brain.
- Degree of awareness during the seizure.
- Level of body movement.
Classifications:
Focal Onset: Retained awareness or impaired awareness; motor or non-motor onset; focal to bilateral tonic-clonic.
Generalized Onset: Motor or non-motor onset seizures.
Unknown Onset: Motor or non-motor or unclassified. Awareness is optional.

Seizures

DEFINITIONS OF SEIZURES

- Seizure—is an abnormal, sudden, excessive, uncontrolled electrical discharge of neurons that occurs in the brain. A seizure may result in alterations in consciousness, motor or sensory ability, or behavior (or any combination).
- Epilepsy—is a chronic disorder with recurrent, unprovoked seizures. Epilepsy may be caused by an abnormality in electrical neuronal activity or an imbalance of neurotransmitters (or both). The term is applied to seizures when the cause is not identifiable or correctable.

TYPES OF SEIZURES

- Generalized seizure—the entire brain is affected.
  - Bilaterally symmetric involving both cerebral hemispheres
  - Convulsive or nonconvulsive; consciousness impaired or lost; tonic-clonic (grand mal); or tonic (tension of muscles); or clonic (repeated bilateral jerking movements)
  - Absence (petit mal)—brief periods of loss of consciousness; blank staring; automatisms
  - Myoclonic—brief jerking or stiffening of extremities
  - Atonic (akinetic)—sudden loss of muscle tone, followed by postictal confusion
- Partial seizure—begins in a specific region of the brain.
  - Focal or local onset
  - Simple partial seizures (unimpaired consciousness, can cause twitching, change in taste or smell)
  - Complex partial seizures (impaired consciousness, unable to respond to questions)
- Unclassified seizure—occurs for no reason and does not fit other categories.

CAUSES OF SEIZURES

- Epilepsy, metabolic disorders, infection, high fever
- Acute alcohol or drug withdrawal, brain trauma, congenital defects
- Electrolyte disturbances, brain tumor, vascular problems

SEIZURE COMPLICATIONS

- Status epilepticus—is a medical emergency during which the patient is in a state of continuous seizure activity. Seizures recur in rapid succession without a return to consciousness between seizures.
- Psychosocial implications—despite improved attitudes and information, epilepsy still carries some social stigma. Patients may experience discrimination in employment and educational opportunities, as well as legal sanctions for driving and operating machinery.

Important nursing implications

Serious/life-threatening implications

Most frequent side effects

Patient teaching

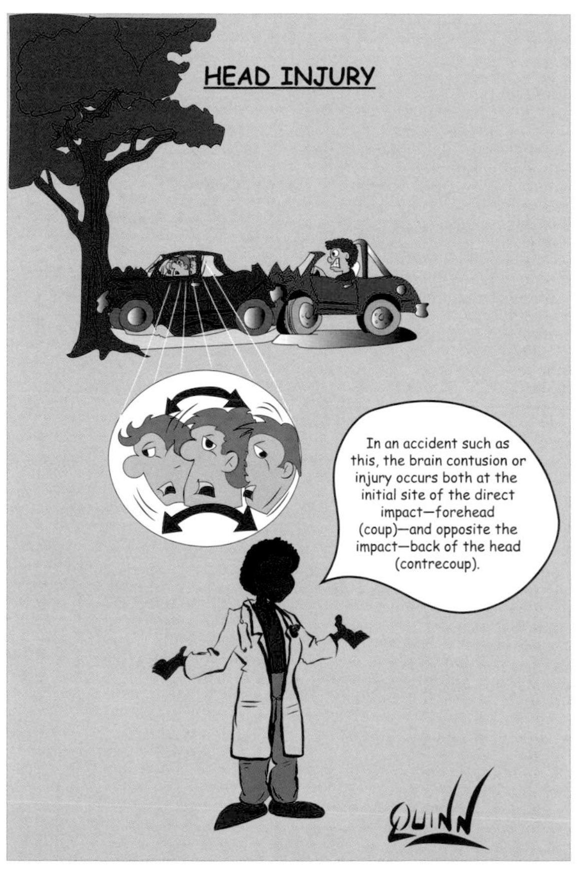
HEAD INJURY
In an accident such as this, the brain contusion or injury occurs both at the initial site of the direct impact—forehead (coup)—and opposite the impact—back of the head (contrecoup).
QUINN

What You Need to Know

Head Injury (Coup and Contrecoup)

TRAUMATIC BRAIN INJURY (TBI)

- External force applied to the head and brain causes a disruption of physiologic stability, locally leading to cerebral contusions and lacerations.
- Increased ICP and potentially dramatic changes in blood flow occur in the brain.
- Diffuse axonal injury (shearing injury) occurs. It is characterized by a decreased loss of consciousness, increased ICP, decerebrate and decorticate posturing, and global cerebral edema.

PRIMARY BRAIN INJURIES

- Closed head injury
  - Blunt trauma has occurred. The skull is not penetrated.
  - Types of closed head injuries:
    - Concussion
    - Diffuse axonal injury
    - Contusion (coup and contrecoup injury): *coup*—direct impact site; *contrecoup*—secondary injury on the opposite side away from injury
- Open head injury
  - Skull fracture or an object penetrates the skull.
  - Depressed fracture—bone is pressed inward into the brain tissue to at least the thickness of the skull.
  - Basilar skull fracture:
    - Occurs at the base of the skull.
    - Results in CSF leakage from the nose or ears.

TYPES OF FORCE

- Acceleration injury—is caused by an external force contacting the head, suddenly placing the head in motion.
- Deceleration injury—occurs when the moving head is suddenly stopped or hits a stationary object.

Important nursing implications | Serious/life-threatening implications

Most frequent side effects | Patient teaching

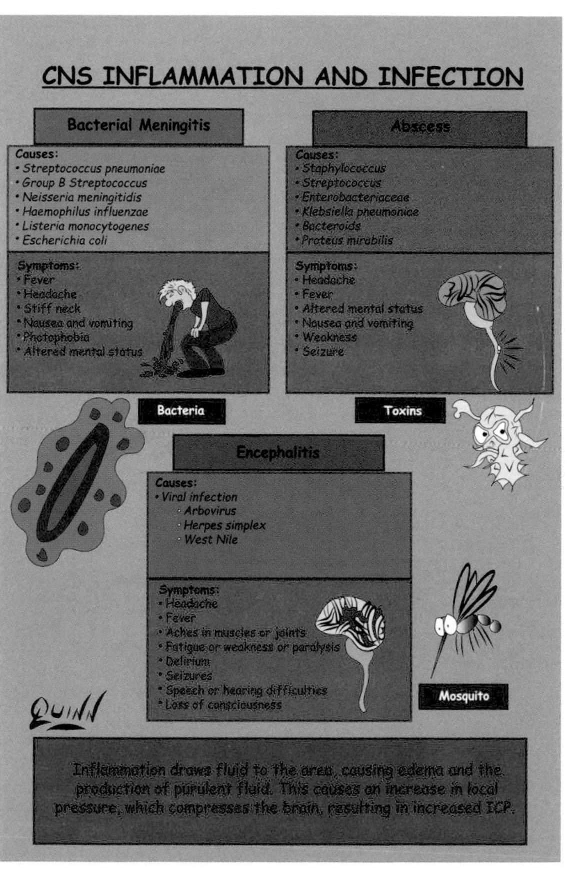
CNS INFLAMMATION AND INFECTION
Bacterial Meningitis
Causes:
• Streptococcus pneumoniae
• Group B Streptococcus
• Neisseria meningitidis
• Haemophilus influenzae
• Listeria monocytogenes
• Escherichia coli
Symptoms:
• Fever
• Headache
• Stiff neck
• Nausea and vomiting
• Photophobia
• Altered mental status
Abscess
Causes:
• Staphylococcus
• Streptococcus
• Enterobacteriaceae
• Klebsiella pneumoniae
• Bacteroids
• Proteus mirabilis
Symptoms:
• Headache
• Fever
• Altered mental status
• Nausea and vomiting
• Weakness
• Seizure
Bacteria
Toxins
Encephalitis
Causes:
• Viral infection
· Arbovirus
· Herpes simplex
· West Nile
Symptoms:
• Headache
• Fever
• Aches in muscles or joints
• Fatigue or weakness or paralysis
• Delirium
• Seizures
• Speech or hearing difficulties
• Loss of consciousness
Mosquito
QUINN
Inflammation draws fluid to the area, causing edema and the production of purulent fluid. This causes an increase in local pressure, which compresses the brain, resulting in increased ICP.

What You Need to Know

CNS Inflammation and Infection

MENINGITIS

- *Meningitis* is an acute inflammation of the arachnoid and pia mater that surrounds the brain and spinal cord, which leads to increased CSF production with a moderate increase in ICP.
- Bacterial meningitis (meningococcal) is considered a medical emergency with a mortality rate of approximately 25%. Viral meningitis is a self-limiting condition.

Signs and Symptoms

- Nuchal rigidity (resistance to flexion of the neck) and positive Kernig and Brudzinski signs
- Headache, nausea, vomiting, and fever
- Photophobia and increased ICP
- Seizure, decreased mental status
- Petechiae rash with meningococcal meningitis

ENCEPHALITIS

- *Encephalitis* is an inflammation of the brain parenchyma and often in the meninges. It affects the cerebrum, brainstem, and cerebellum. Hemorrhage, edema, and necrosis occur in cerebral hemispheres. Encephalitis differs from meningitis because cerebral function changes; it remains normal with meningitis.
- Viral cause—Herpes simplex; West Nile virus; Arbovirus (mosquitoes are often the vectors).

Signs and Symptoms

- Nonspecific fever, headache, nausea, vomiting
- Altered cerebral functioning—altered mental status, delirium, motor or sensory deficits (weakness to paralysis); seizures
- Muscle and joint aches, fatigue

BRAIN ABSCESS

- *Brain abscess* is a purulent infection of the brain with pus forming in the extradural, subdural, or intracerebral area of the brain.
- Is the result of a local or systemic infection (e.g., ear, tooth or sinus, bacterial endocarditis, skull fracture).

Signs and Symptoms

- Findings may be atypical at presentation, but often include increased ICP and focal symptoms.
- May include: headache, fever, altered mental status, weakness, nausea, and vomiting.

Important nursing implications | Serious/life-threatening implications
Most frequent side effects | Patient teaching

CNS DEGENERATIVE DISEASES

Parkinson Disease	Multiple Sclerosis (MS)
Degenerative disorder of the basal ganglia that involves loss of dopaminergic pigmented neurons.	Diffuse, progressive, chronic inflammatory, demyelinating, autoimmune disorder of the CNS.
Motor • Tremor at rest • Rigidity, cogwheel • Akinesia/bradykinesia • Postural instability **Nonmotor** • Masklike expression • Fatigue	• Periods of remission and exacerbation • Progressive paresthesia and weakness • Visual disturbances • Cerebellar incoordination • Urinary dysfunction

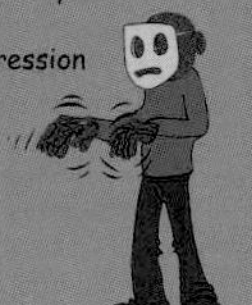

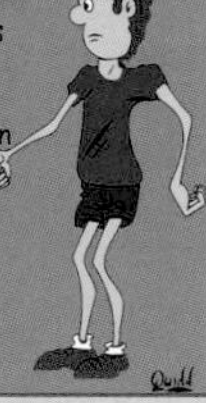

Guillain-Barré Syndrome	Myasthenia Gravis
Demyelinating disorder caused by an immunologic reaction directed at the peripheral nerves.	Chronic autoimmune disorder that is antibody-mediated acting on the neuromuscular junction.
• Ascending flaccid paresis • Respiratory insufficiency • Autonomic nervous system instability • Areflexia	• Insidious onset • Diplopia, ptosis, and ocular palsies • Difficulty chewing and swallowing • Muscle fatigue and weakness • Expressionless

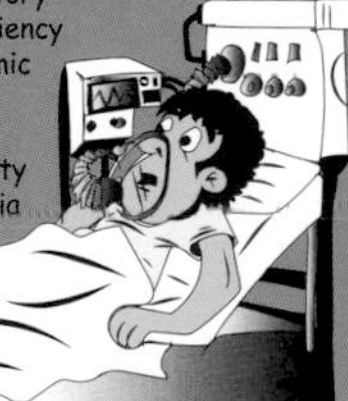

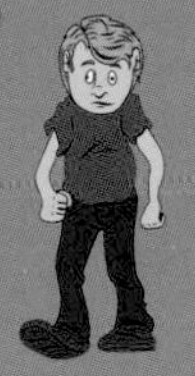

What You Need to Know

CNS Degenerative Diseases

PARKINSON DISEASE

- *Parkinson disease* is characterized by an insidious and gradual progression. A degenerative disorder of the basal ganglia.

Signs and Symptoms

- Use the mnemonic TRAP to remember hallmark signs: **T**remor at rest; **R**igidity (cogwheel); **A**kinesia; **P**ostural instability (shuffling gait). A slight tremor at first that is more prominent at rest, pill-rolling tremor, changes in voluntary movement (akinesia/bradykinesia—slowing down in initiation and execution of movement), problems with manual dexterity, and shuffling gait are all primary symptoms.
- Other symptoms include fatigue, changes in facial expression (masklike), uncontrolled drooling, dementia, and orthostatic hypotension.

MULTIPLE SCLEROSIS

- *Multiple sclerosis*, an autoimmune disorder, is characterized by periods of remission and exacerbation with chronic inflammation and demyelination (patchy areas of plaque in the white matter). Symptoms depend on the CNS nerves affected.
- Onset is insidious and gradual.

Signs and Symptoms

- Progressive paresthesia (numbness, tingling, or burning) and weakness. Flexor spasms at night, intention tremor, bowel and bladder dysfunction.
- Scanning speech, blurred vision, diplopia, decreased visual acuity, scotomas, nystagmus.

GUILLAIN-BARRÉ SYNDROME

- *Guillain-Barré syndrome* is characterized by an immune system that starts to destroy the myelin sheath that surrounds the axons at the peripheral nerves; this destruction is the most common clinical pattern.

Signs and Symptoms

- Muscle weakness and pain have an abrupt onset. Ascending flaccid paresis with weakness and paresthesia beginning in the lower extremities and progressing upward.
- Cerebral function or pupillary signs are not affected.
- Ineffective breathing pattern occurs as a result of ascending paralysis.

MYASTHENIA GRAVIS

- *Myasthenia Gravis* is a chronic autoimmune disorder that is antibody mediated with an insidious onset.

Signs and Symptoms

Progressive paresis of affected muscle groups. Involvement of upper and lower respiratory system causes chewing, swallowing, and breathing difficulties; involvement of eye muscles causes ptosis, diplopia, and ocular palsies.

Important nursing implications	Serious/life-threatening implications
Most frequent side effects	Patient teaching

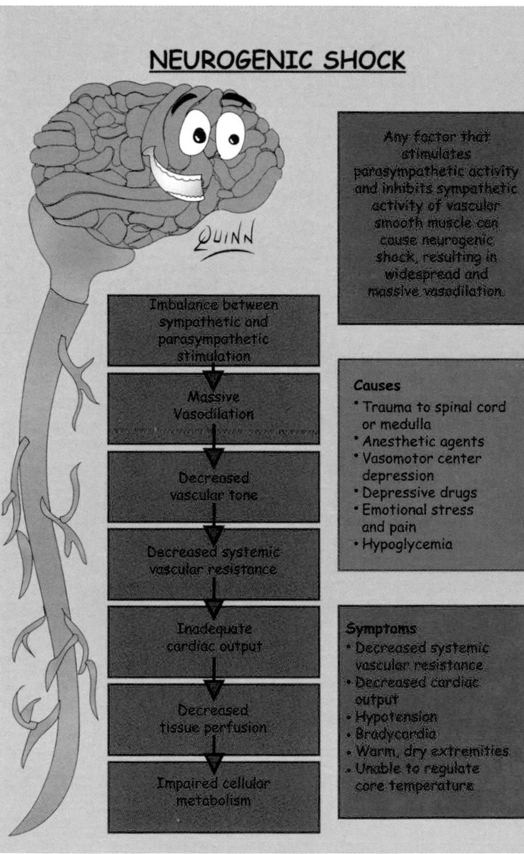
NEUROGENIC SHOCK
QUINN
Any factor that stimulates parasympathetic activity and inhibits sympathetic activity of vascular smooth muscle can cause neurogenic shock, resulting in widespread and massive vasodilation.
Imbalance between sympathetic and parasympathetic stimulation
Massive Vasodilation
Decreased vascular tone
Decreased systemic vascular resistance
Inadequate cardiac output
Decreased tissue perfusion
Impaired cellular metabolism
Causes
• Trauma to spinal cord or medulla
• Anesthetic agents
• Vasomotor center depression
• Depressive drugs
• Emotional stress and pain
• Hypoglycemia
Symptoms
• Decreased systemic vascular resistance
• Decreased cardiac output
• Hypotension
• Bradycardia
• Warm, dry extremities
• Unable to regulate core temperature

What You Need to Know

Neurogenic Shock

SIGNIFICANCE OF NEUROGENIC SHOCK

Neurogenic shock (also called *vasogenic shock*) occurs when widespread and massive vasodilation develops, which is the result of an imbalance between the parasympathetic and sympathetic nervous systems. This imbalance occurs after a spinal cord injury at the fifth thoracic (T5) vertebra or above.

Although spinal shock and neurogenic shock can occur in the same patient, these two disorders are not the same. *Spinal shock* occurs after spinal cord injury and is characterized by flaccid paralysis below the level of lesion, along with loss of reflex activity and bowel and bladder function.

PRECIPITATING FACTORS

- Hemodynamic consequence of an injury or disease to the spinal cord at T5 or higher or both
- Spinal anesthesia
- Vasomotor center depression (severe pain, drugs, hypoglycemia, injury)

Signs and Symptoms

- Hypotension from massive vasodilation and bradycardia from unopposed activation of the parasympathetic nervous system
- Decreased systemic vascular resistance (SVR); decreased cardiac output (CO); decreased central venous pressure (CVP)
- Difficulty with core temperature regulation caused by hypothalamic dysfunction
- Decreased skin perfusion (patient takes on the temperature of the environment—poikilothermia); cool or warm, dry

Treatment

- Symptomatically directed by restoring fluids to the circulating blood volume

---

Important nursing implications | Serious/life-threatening implications

Most frequent side effects | Patient teaching

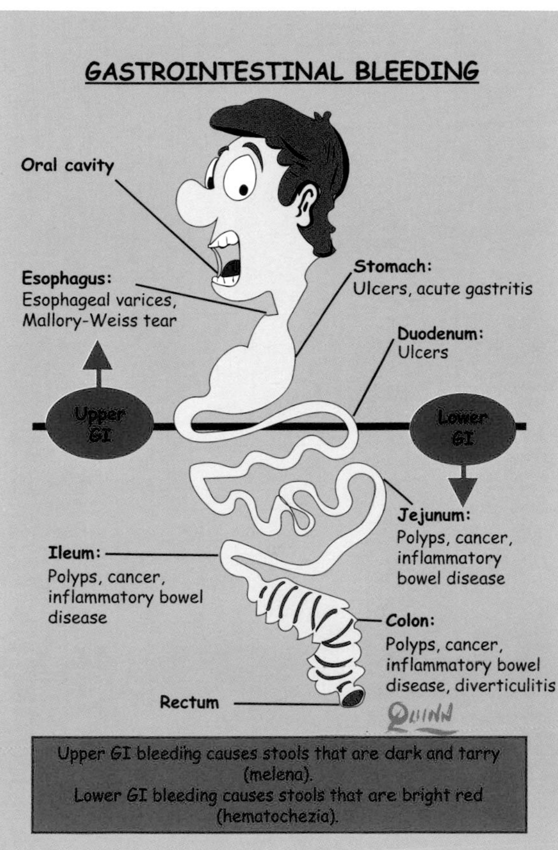
GASTROINTESTINAL BLEEDING
Oral cavity
Esophagus:
Esophageal varices, Mallory-Weiss tear
Stomach:
Ulcers, acute gastritis
Duodenum:
Ulcers
Upper GI
Lower GI
Jejunum:
Polyps, cancer, inflammatory bowel disease
Ileum:
Polyps, cancer, inflammatory bowel disease
Colon:
Polyps, cancer, inflammatory bowel disease, diverticulitis
Rectum
Upper GI bleeding causes stools that are dark and tarry (melena).
Lower GI bleeding causes stools that are bright red (hematochezia).

What You Need to Know

Gastrointestinal Bleeding

SIGNIFICANCE OF GASTROINTESTINAL BLEEDING

The overall effect of gastrointestinal (GI) bleeding depends on the amount of blood lost over a specific period, an individual's age, associated conditions, and the effectiveness of the treatment.

- Blood urea nitrogen (BUN) will increase if the blood has been digested (e.g., GI hemorhhage). The breakdown of red blood cells (RBCs) produces an increased amount of protein, which increases the BUN.
- When plasma volume is rapidly lost, the replacement plasma does not immediately occur, which is why hemoglobin and hematocrit are not good indicators of immediate blood loss.
- Because hematocrit is the percentage of plasma occupied by the RBCs, the loss of RBCs may not be reflected for 24 hours.
- Hemorrhage is the most serious complication of GI bleeding and tends to occur more in patients with gastric ulcers and older adults.

CAUSES OF GASTROINTESTINAL BLEEDING

- **Upper GI bleeding** can be caused from (1) ulcers in the esophagus, stomach, or duodenum; (2) esophageal varices from portal hypertension; or (3) gastric tears from a malignancy.
- **Lower GI bleeding** can be caused from ulcers or polyps in the jejunum, ileum, colon, or rectum, as well as from inflammatory bowel disease, diverticulitis, cancer, or hemorrhoids.

SIGNS AND SYMPTOMS

- **Melena**, or black tarry stools, indicates that the digestive process has broken down the blood, usually a sign of upper GIB.
- **Hematochezia** is fresh blood passing from the rectum, usually a sign of lower GIB.
- **Occult bleeding**, or trace amounts of blood occurring in an apparently normal stool, is determined by a guaiac test on the stool. Over time, occult bleeding may cause anemia.

Important nursing implications | Serious/life-threatening implications

Most frequent side effects | Patient teaching

ABDOMINAL DISTENTION

CAUSES
Irritable bowel syndrome
Constipation
Obstruction
Peritonitis (fluid)
Adhesions
Tumor
Obesity
Hypomotility
Intussception
Acute abdomen (appendicitis; cholecystitis)

My stomach is so stretched out and tight. I feel nauseous from being so full of air.
QUINN

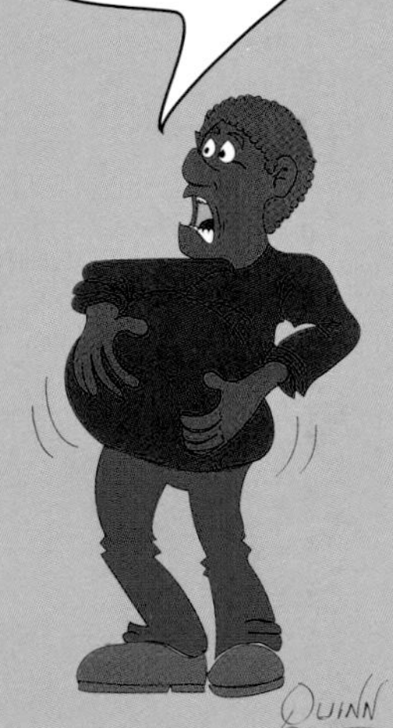

The cause is usually in the lower GI tract. Nausea and vomiting are common problems.

What You Need to Know

Abdominal Distention

ASSESSMENT

The abdomen is divided into four quadrants to facilitate a description of the findings. One imaginary line is drawn horizontally, and another drawn vertically across the umbilicus, dividing the abdomen into four quadrants—upper and lower right quadrants and upper and lower left quadrants. Abdomen distention may cause nausea and vomiting.

Inspection

The abdomen should be observed for any masses. It should not appear to be full or distended. Gases, tumors, or fluid in the abdomen will make the abdomen appear distended.

Auscultation

Bowel sounds should be auscultated in all four quadrants. Normally, bowel sounds will occur five or more times a minute. Gurgling can be heard every 5–20 s with a normal frequency of 5–30 per minute. Distention may decrease or increase bowel sounds.

Palpation

The abdomen should be soft to palpation without any specific areas of tenderness.

Percussion

Normally, the upper left quadrant will sound hollow or tympanic, indicating underlying air. With distention secondary to air, the hollow sound may be percussed over the other quadrants as well. Distention caused by retained feces will sound dull with little resonance, especially in the lower left quadrant.

CAUSES

The following conditions may cause abdominal distention:

- Reaction to food intake, causing increased gas production, irritable bowel disease
- Blockage (e.g., tumor, volvulus, adhesions, ileus, incarcerated hernia) in the intestine, preventing passage of gas and GI contents or constipation with retained feces
- Inflammation in the abdomen—inflammatory bowel disease, peritonitis, cholecystitis
- Increased size of the liver with development of ascites
- Hemorrhage into the abdomen from perforated ulcers or tumors

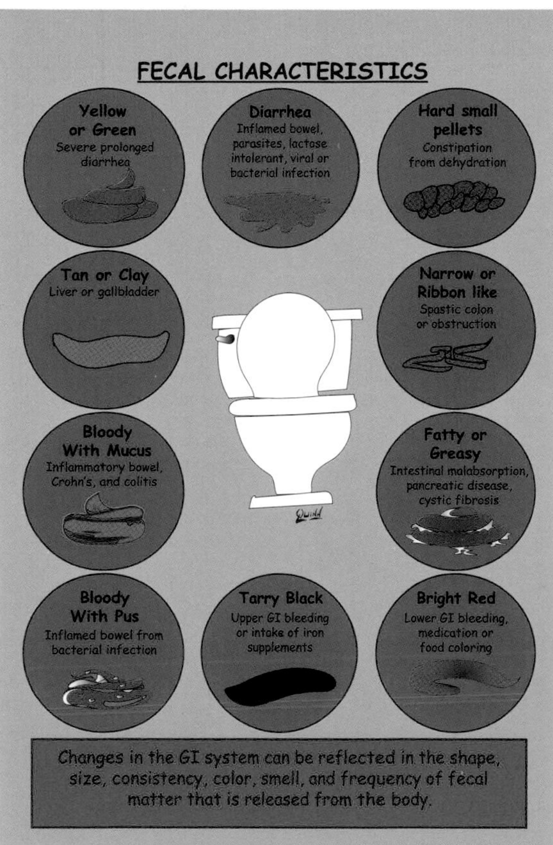
FECAL CHARACTERISTICS
Yellow or Green
Severe prolonged diarrhea
Diarrhea
Inflamed bowel, parasites, lactose intolerant, viral or bacterial infection
Hard small pellets
Constipation from dehydration
Tan or Clay
Liver or gallbladder
Narrow or Ribbon like
Spastic colon or obstruction
Bloody With Mucus
Inflammatory bowel, Crohn's, and colitis
Fatty or Greasy
Intestinal malabsorption, pancreatic disease, cystic fibrosis
Bloody With Pus
Inflamed bowel from bacterial infection
Tarry Black
Upper GI bleeding or intake of iron supplements
Bright Red
Lower GI bleeding, medication or food coloring
Changes in the GI system can be reflected in the shape, size, consistency, color, smell, and frequency of fecal matter that is released from the body.

What You Need to Know

Fecal Characteristics

NORMAL FECAL CHARACTERISTICS

- Color is usually brown, the odor is dependent on food intake, and the form is soft.
- Bowel movements may occur daily or two to three times a week, depending on intake. The shape should resemble the diameter of the rectum.

ABNORMAL FECAL CHARACTERISTICS

Shape

- Narrow or ribbonlike stool may reflect an obstruction in the lower GI tract.

Consistency

- Diarrhea or liquid stool may occur from infection or with intake of some antibiotics. Consistent, frequent diarrhea may cause significant fluid and electrolyte loss.
- Hard small pellet like stool is indicative of constipation, which is generally caused by dehydration.

COLOR

Bloody Stool (Hematochezia)

- Bright red bloody stools may occur with lower GI bleeding. Commonly caused by hemorrhoids, but may be indicative of colon cancer or a ruptured diverticulum.
- Stool that is bloody with mucus usually indicates inflammatory bowel disease, Crohn's disease, or colitis.
- Stool that is bloody with pus is characteristic of a bacterial infection.

Black Tarry Stool (Melena)

- May occur with bleeding in the upper GI tract.
- Blood has been acted on by the digestive enzymes and turns very black and sticky. It has a strong characteristic odor.
- Black stools also occur with increased iron intake or medications (e.g., bismuth subsalicylate).

Clay-Colored Stool

- Light, tan-colored stool may be indicative of gallbladder or liver disease. A decrease in conjugated bilirubin (bile) causes the light color.

Frothy, Fatty Stool (Steatorrhea)

- Occurs when problems with fat digestion are present.
- Is commonly observed in children with cystic fibrosis or in adults with pancreatic disease or cholecystitis.
- Indicates malabsorption or a loss of bile, which is necessary for adequate fat digestion.

Important nursing implications

Serious/life-threatening implications

Most frequent side effects

Patient teaching

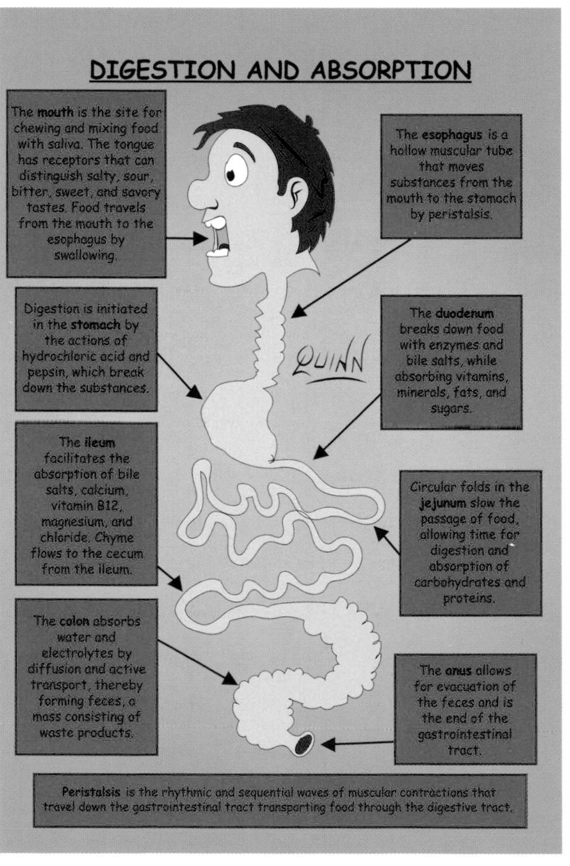
DIGESTION AND ABSORPTION
The **mouth** is the site for chewing and mixing food with saliva. The tongue has receptors that can distinguish salty, sour, bitter, sweet, and savory tastes. Food travels from the mouth to the esophagus by swallowing.
The **esophagus** is a hollow muscular tube that moves substances from the mouth to the stomach by peristalsis.
Digestion is initiated in the **stomach** by the actions of hydrochloric acid and pepsin, which break down the substances.
QUINN
The **duodenum** breaks down food with enzymes and bile salts, while absorbing vitamins, minerals, fats, and sugars.
The **ileum** facilitates the absorption of bile salts, calcium, vitamin B12, magnesium, and chloride. Chyme flows to the cecum from the ileum.
Circular folds in the **jejunum** slow the passage of food, allowing time for digestion and absorption of carbohydrates and proteins.
The **colon** absorbs water and electrolytes by diffusion and active transport, thereby forming feces, a mass consisting of waste products.
The **anus** allows for evacuation of the feces and is the end of the gastrointestinal tract.
Peristalsis is the rhythmic and sequential waves of muscular contractions that travel down the gastrointestinal tract transporting food through the digestive tract.

What You Need to Know

Digestion and Absorption

MOUTH

- Breaks down the food and mixes it with saliva to initiate the digestive process. Salivary glands secrete amylase, which begins the digestion of carbohydrates.

ESOPHAGUS AND ESOPHAGEAL SPHINCTERS

- The esophagus moves substances from the mouth to the stomach.
- The upper sphincter prevents air from entering the stomach, while the lower esophageal sphincter (LES) prevents regurgitation of food mass into the esophagus.

STOMACH

- Secretes pepsinogen, gastrin, and hydrochloric acid (HCl) that mix with the food to form chyme.
- Intrinsic factor is also secreted in the stomach, which provides for the absorption of vitamin B12 in the small intestine (ileum).
- No nutrients are absorbed in the stomach.

SMALL INTESTINE—DUODENUM, JEJUNUM, ILEUM

- Small intestine begins at the pyloric valve and goes to the ileocecal valve, which empties into the cecum of the colon.
- Duodenum mixes the chyme with intestinal enzymes, pancreatic enzymes, and bile salts to breakdown carbohydrates into simple sugars, proteins into amino acids, and fats into fatty acids and monoglycerides.
- Jejunum slows the passage of food to allow time for digestion and absorption.
- Ileum facilitates absorption of bile salts, calcium, vitamin B12, magnesium, and chloride.
- As chyme is moved through the small intestine, it is exposed to a large amount of intestinal mucosa, where the nutrients are actually absorbed.
- All nutrients from food intake are absorbed in the small intestine.
- Approximately 85% of water and fluid intake is also absorbed in the small intestine.

COLON

- Cecum pouch connects the large intestine to the small intestine, which is where the appendix is located.
- Is divided into four sections: (1) ascending, (2) transverse, (3) descending, and (4) sigmoid, which terminates at the rectum.
- Serves as a reservoir for fecal mass and absorbs water and electrolytes.
- No absorption of nutrients occurs.

Important nursing implications | Serious/life-threatening implications
Most frequent side effects | Patient teaching

MALABSORPTION

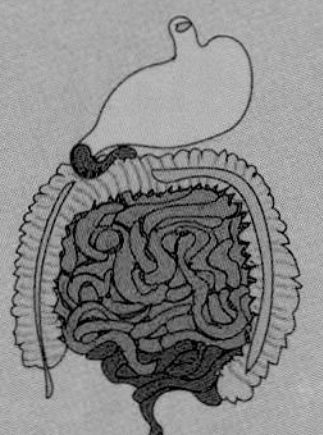

GI System

Common Causes:
- Infection
- Medications
- Cystic fibrosis
- Chronic pancreatitis
- Celiac disease
- Lactose intolerance
- Parasite infection
- Small intestine surgery

Symptoms:
- Weight loss
- Gas and bloating
- Stomach cramping
- Diarrhea
- Steatorrhea
- Weakness and fatigue

Malabsorption is the inability to absorb nutrients, vitamins, and minerals from the intestinal tract.

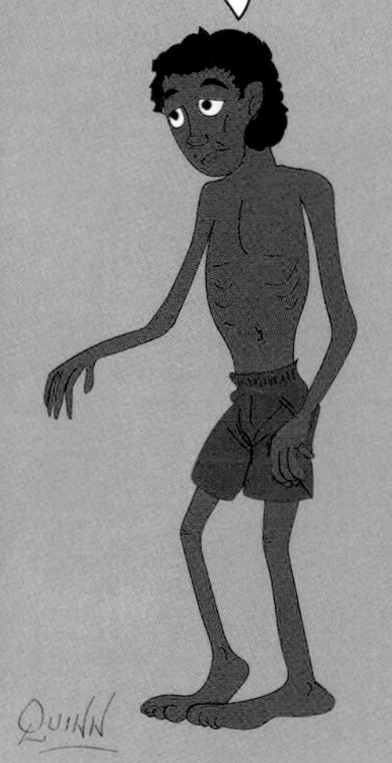

What You Need to Know

Malabsorption

SIGNIFICANCE OF MALABSORPTION

- Malabsorption occurs when the digested nutrients are not absorbed or transported across the intestinal mucosa.
  - Signs and symptoms include: chronic diarrhea (classic symptom), unintentional weight loss, gas, bloating, flatus, stomach cramping, steatorrhea, weakness, and fatigue.
- Malnutrition is a deficit or an imbalance in the dietary intake.

COMMON CAUSES

Celiac (Gluten Sensitive-Enteropathy)

- Immune disease that affects the absorption of gluten found in wheat, barley, rye, and oats.

Enzyme Deficiencies

- Pancreatic—is primarily a lack of pancreatic enzymes (e.g., lipase) that are necessary for fat digestion.
- Lactase—is a congenital defect in which a lack of lactase exists to facilitate the digestion of milk and milk products.
- Bile salt—is the lack of conjugated bile salts, which are necessary for fat digestion.

Inflammatory Bowel Disease

- Process destroys sections of the normal mucosa of the small intestine.
- Inflammation can be either ulcerative colitis or Crohn's disease.
- Diarrhea and poor nutrition are common with both conditions.

Bacteria

- Microorganisms harbored in the small intestine may destroy or inhibit the absorption of vitamin B12.

Short Bowel Syndrome

- Condition where the body is unable to absorb enough nutrients from the foods ingested.
- May occur from extensive resection of the small intestine.

Interference With Blood Flow Through the Mesenteric or Celiac Arteries

- Intestinal and gastric surgery along with radiation enteritis results in malabsorption.

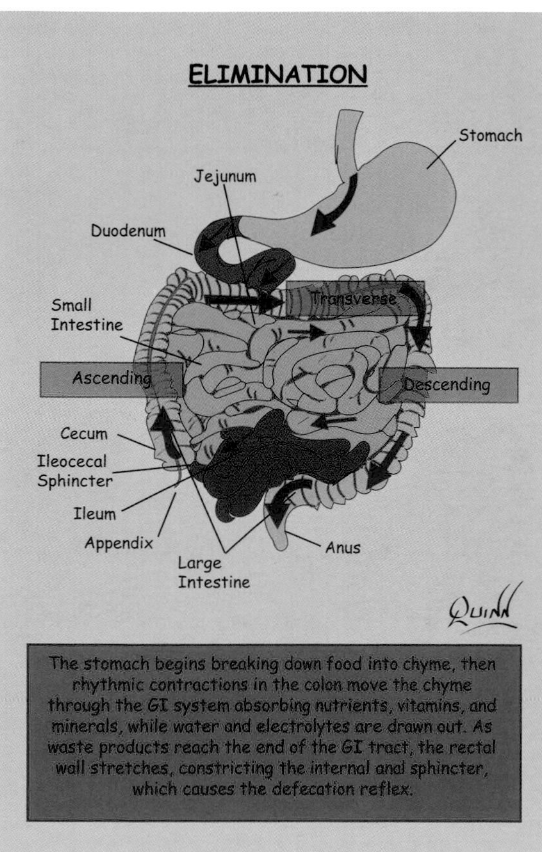
ELIMINATION
Stomach
Jejunum
Duodenum
Small Intestine
Transverse
Ascending
Descending
Cecum
Ileocecal Sphincter
Ileum
Appendix
Large Intestine
Anus
Quinn
The stomach begins breaking down food into chyme, then rhythmic contractions in the colon move the chyme through the GI system absorbing nutrients, vitamins, and minerals, while water and electrolytes are drawn out. As waste products reach the end of the GI tract, the rectal wall stretches, constricting the internal anal sphincter, which causes the defecation reflex.

What You Need to Know

Elimination

LARGE INTESTINE

- Is approximately 5–6 feet long and consists of several sections.
  - *Cecum* receives chyme from the ileum of the small intestine. The appendix is attached to the cecum. The cecum empties into the *ascending portion* of the large intestine.
  - *Transverse portion* of the large intestine moves the fecal mass across the upper portion of the abdomen to the *descending colon* on the left side.
  - From the descending colon, feces travel through the *sigmoid colon* into the rectum.
- Large intestine secretes mucus from the goblet cells.
- Primary function is to absorb water and electrolytes (e.g., sodium, chloride).

VAGUS AND PARASYMPATHETIC NERVES

- Innervate the large intestine and initiate the stimulus to propel the movement of feces through the intestine.
- Blood supply to the large intestine is primarily from branches of the inferior and superior mesenteric arteries.
- Any decrease or ischemia in these vessels will affect the function of the large intestine.

GASTROCOLONIC REFLEX

- Occurs immediately after eating when chyme enters the cecum, and the fecal mass is propelled through the colon.
- Movement of feces into the sigmoid colon, which initiates the defecation reflex.
- Increased intraabdominal pressure facilitates defecation.

VALSALVA MANEUVER

- Is accomplished by inhaling and forcing the diaphragm and chest movement against a closed glottis.
- Causes an increase in intrathoracic pressure and intraabdominal pressure, which is transmitted to the rectum.
- Initiation of this maneuver is contraindicated in patients with cardiac problems, eye surgery, abdominal surgery, or head injury.

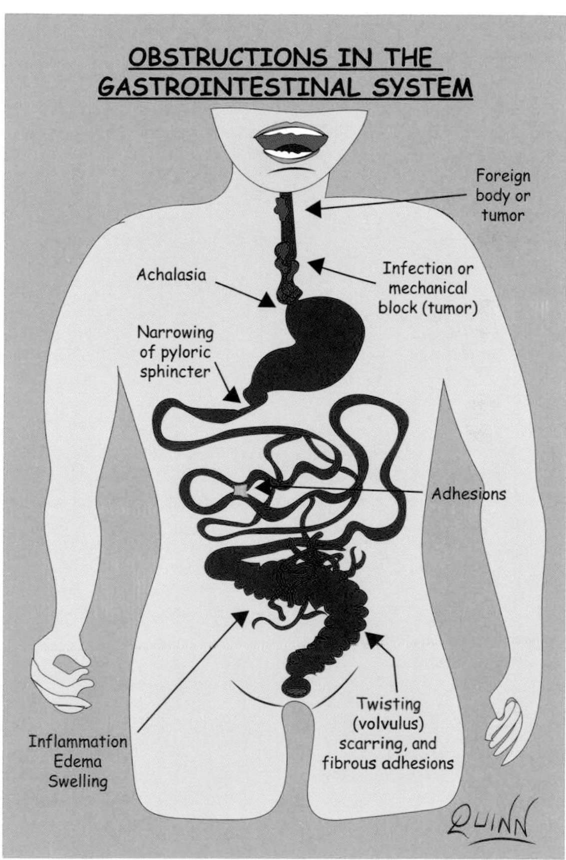
OBSTRUCTIONS IN THE GASTROINTESTINAL SYSTEM
Foreign body or tumor
Achalasia
Infection or mechanical block (tumor)
Narrowing of pyloric sphincter
Adhesions
Inflammation Edema Swelling
Twisting (volvulus) scarring, and fibrous adhesions
QUINN

What You Need to Know

Obstructions in the Gastrointestinal System

TYPES OF OBSTRUCTION

Mechanical Obstruction

- Occlusion or obstruction has occurred in the GI tract.
- Adhesions, tumors, hernias, or foreign bodies can cause the obstruction.

Neuromuscular Obstruction

- Area of the GI tract lacks adequate innervation to propel food or nutrients.
- Paralytic ileus and congenital megacolon are examples.

Vascular Disorders

- Obstruction of adequate blood flow may occur with mesenteric artery infarctions.

CAUSES OF OBSTRUCTIONS

The onset of the obstruction, either rapid or gradual, and the location and amount of intestine involved dictate the course of the problem. The higher the obstruction in the intestinal tract, the faster the symptoms will be expressed.

Dysphagia

- Mechanical obstruction of the esophagus causes difficulty in swallowing.
- Achalasia occurs secondary to a decrease in innervation to the middle or lower portions of the esophagus.

Hernia

- Portion of the intestine protrudes through the abdominal wall.
- If the hernia is strangulated, then an intestinal or a vascular obstruction is present.

Intussusception

- The telescoping of the bowel, which may cause vascular obstruction.

Volvulus

- A twisting of the intestine, more common in the large intestine.

Diverticulosis

- Is an outpouching of the colon.
- Inflammation (diverticulitis) may cause a mechanical obstruction.

Tumor

- Growth develops into the intestinal lumen.

- Colorectal cancers are the most common and treatable GI cancers and occur more in patients over 60 years of age.

Paralytic Ileus

- Loss of peristaltic activity occurs in the intestine.
- May be associated with abdominal surgery, narcotics, peritonitis, or states of immobility.

Fibrous Adhesions and Scarring

- Adhesions and scarring are due to abdominal surgery, trauma, or peritonitis.

Important nursing implications

Serious/life-threatening implications

Most frequent side effects

Patient teaching

COMMON SYMPTOMS OF HEPATIC AND BILIARY PROBLEMS

Hepatitis causes hepatocelluar jaundice because the liver can't metabolize bilirubin.

Cholecystitis is an inflamed gallbladder. Cholelithiasis is the formation of a gallstone.

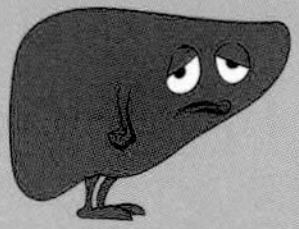

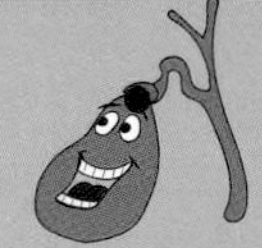

Liver

Gallbladder

The liver parenchymal cells are destroyed in cirrhosis because of alcohol or infection.

Cholelithiasis may impede bile flow causing obstructive jaundice.

Symptoms caused by obstructed bile flow:

- Jaundice
- Pruritus
- Steatorrhea
- Clay colored stool
- Dark amber urine
- Intolerance of fatty foods
- Bleeding

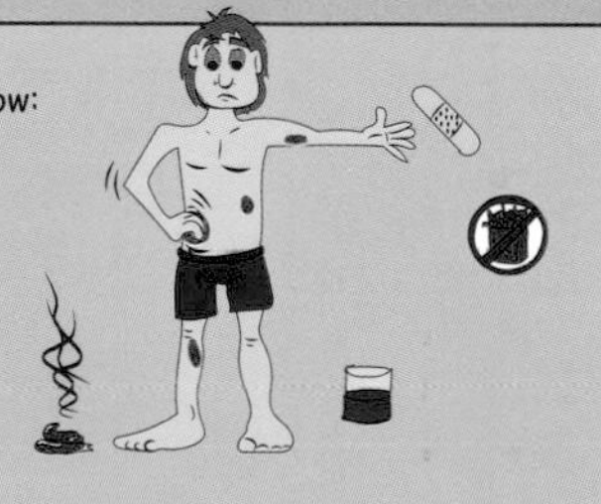

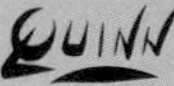

What You Need to Know

Common Symptoms of Hepatic and Biliary Problems

HEPATITIS

Hepatitis is caused by a virus that attacks the liver. Regardless of the type of virus, the effects are similar. Jaundice is a common occurrence as a result of biliary stasis.

Signs and Symptoms

- Fatigue, anorexia, nausea and vomiting, malaise, headache
- Jaundice and abdominal pain, followed by recovery

CIRRHOSIS

Cirrhosis is a progressive deterioration of the liver cells. The liver attempts to regenerate damaged cells but most often is unsuccessful. Cirrhosis may be caused by excessive alcohol intake, biliary obstruction, or chronic right-sided heart failure. It may also occur secondary to the complications of hepatitis.

Signs and Symptoms

- Generally slow onset
- Anorexia, dyspepsia, flatulence, nausea, and vomiting
- Diarrhea or constipation, general abdominal discomfort
- Jaundice, skin lesions (spider angiomas)
- Hematologic problems (thrombocytopenia, anemia, coagulation disorders)
- Endocrine problems (imbalance of adrenocortical hormones, retention of sodium and water, potassium loss from failure to metabolize aldosterone)
- Peripheral neuropathy, most often from dietary deficiencies

Complications may include portal hypertension, ascites, or hepatic encephalopathy.

CHOLECYSTITIS

Cholecystitis is an inflammation of the gallbladder. Most often the cause is cholelithiasis or the presence of gallstones that obstruct the flow of bile. Inflammation may also occur in older adults in the absence of gallstones.

Signs and Symptoms

- Pain may be in the upper right quadrant or may radiate to the upper middle back.
- Fever and jaundice are common, and symptoms may occur after ingesting a meal high in fat.
- Obstructed bile flow may cause pruritus, dark amber urine, steatorrhea, or clay colored stool.

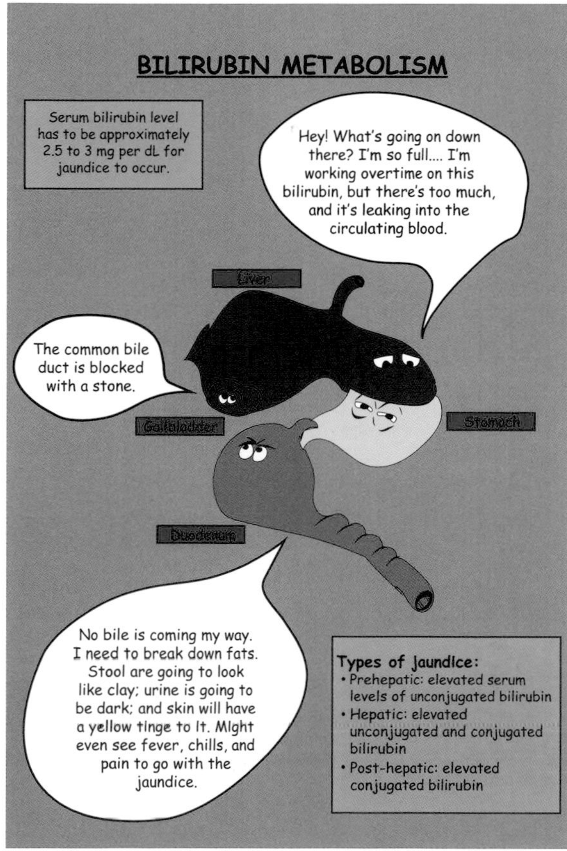
BILIRUBIN METABOLISM
Serum bilirubin level has to be approximately 2.5 to 3 mg per dL for jaundice to occur.
Hey! What's going on down there? I'm so full.... I'm working overtime on this bilirubin, but there's too much, and it's leaking into the circulating blood.
Liver
The common bile duct is blocked with a stone.
Gallbladder
Stomach
Duodenum
No bile is coming my way. I need to break down fats. Stool are going to look like clay; urine is going to be dark; and skin will have a yellow tinge to It. MIght even see fever, chills, and pain to go with the jaundice.
Types of Jaundice:
• Prehepatic: elevated serum levels of unconjugated bilirubin
• Hepatic: elevated unconjugated and conjugated bilirubin
• Post-hepatic: elevated conjugated bilirubin

What You Need to Know

Bilirubin Metabolism

SIGNIFICANCE OF BILIRUBIN

Bilirubin is the byproduct of the breakdown of red blood cells (RBCs), which are known as erythrocytes. The macrophages in the liver and the spleen break down the RBCs. The Kupffer cells in the liver separate the hemoglobin or heme component from the globin component. The heme is then converted into iron to be stored in the liver, and the byproduct is converted to bilirubin. Increased levels of bilirubin are present when a bile duct obstruction is present or if liver disease has developed.

Unconjugated bilirubin is a waste product of RBC taken up by the liver and is converted into conjugated bilirubin. It is not soluble in water and is bound to plasma protein.

Conjugated bilirubin—is water-soluble and is excreted into the bile to be cleared from the body. Bile contains bile salts, which are necessary for fat breakdown and digestion.

BILIRUBIN LEVELS

- **Indirect (unconjugated)** is less than 0.8 mg/dL and increases with hemolysis of RBCs.
- **Direct (conjugated)** is less than 0.3 mg/dL and increases with liver damage from bile obstruction.
- **Total bilirubin**—is less than 1.2 mg/dL and increases with biliary obstruction.
- **Urobilinogen**—conjugated bilirubin is present in the ileum and colon and is excreted in the feces.

JAUNDICE

- Occurs either from a problem in the normal metabolism of bilirubin or from a problem with the flow of bile into the liver or gallbladder. Jaundice usually becomes evident when the total serum bilirubin is greater than 2.5 mg/dL.
- **Physiologic jaundice of the newborn**—occurs with an immature liver and poor conjugation of bilirubin and is a normal process.
- **Hemolytic jaundice**—breakdown of RBCs is associated with transfusion reaction, sickle cell crisis, or hemolytic anemia.
- **Hepatocellular jaundice**—liver is unable to pick the bilirubin from the blood or conjugate it or excrete it.

- **Obstructive jaundice**—may be intrahepatic or extrahepatic and is caused by an obstruction (gallstones, tumor, inflammation).

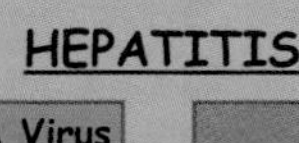

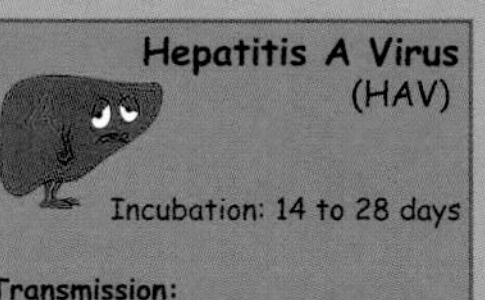

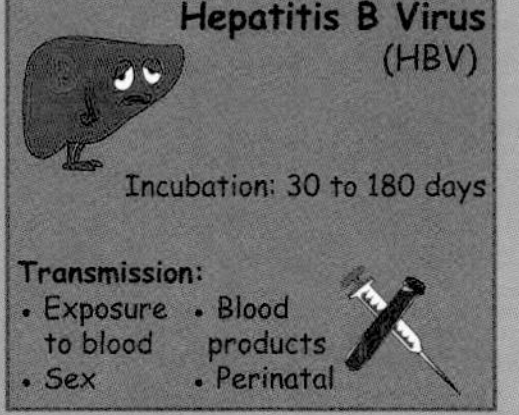

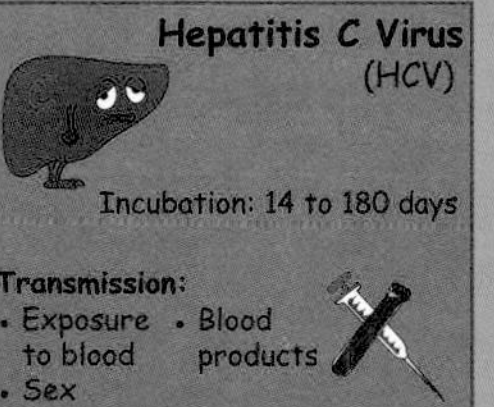

QUINN

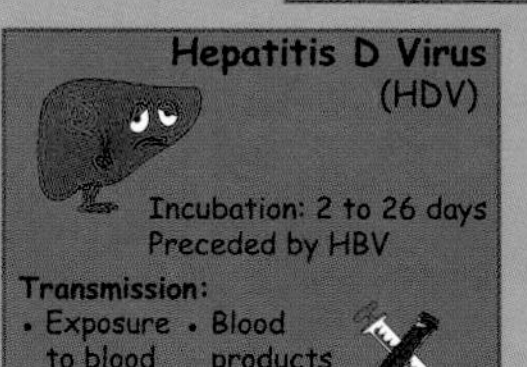

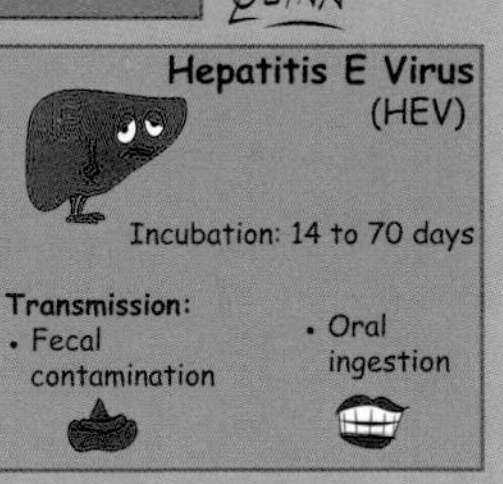

Hepatitis has three phases: prodomal, icteric, and recovery.

What You Need to Know

Hepatitis

SIGNIFICANCE OF HEPATITIS

Hepatitis is a viral infection causing inflammation and necrosis of liver cells.

SIGNS AND SYMPTOMS

- Symptoms are very similar among all types, but the overall severity depends on the individual's age, state of health, and type of the infecting virus.
- All individuals with a history of hepatitis should not donate blood or drink alcohol.

TYPES OF HEPATITIS

- Hepatitis A (HAV) transmission through fecal contamination and oral ingestion
- Hepatitis B (HBV) transmission through blood, sexual intercourse, and perinatal
- Hepatitis C (HDV) transmission through blood and sexual intercourse
- Hepatitis D (HDV) transmission through blood, blood with HBV, and sexual intercourse
- Hepatitis E (HEV) transmission through fecal contamination and oral ingestion

PHASES OF HEPATITIS

Prodromal

- Occurs before the occurrence of jaundice.
- Is characterized by fatigue, anorexia, nausea and vomiting, and low-grade fever.
- Onset is usually approximately 2 weeks after exposure.

Icteric

- Jaundice (hepatocellular) occurs secondary to biliary stasis.
- Urine is dark, liver is enlarged, fatigue and abdominal pain are present.
- Serum bilirubin levels increase, and prothrombin time may be prolonged.

Recovery (Posticteric)

- After resolution of jaundice, the liver may remain enlarged and tender.
- Results of liver function testing generally returns to normal.

ALTERATIONS IN RENAL AND URINARY FUNCTION

My system is blocked. Things are going to back up.

Obstruction:

- Renal calculus
- Neurogenic bladder
- Tumor

I can't filter if I'm inflamed or infected.

Infection:

- Cystitis
- Pyelonephritis

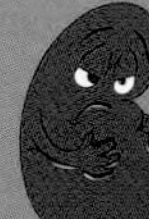

My antigens and antibodies are affecting my filtration.

Glomerular disorders:

- Glomerulonephritis
- Nephrotic syndrome
- Nephritic syndrome

I'm in real trouble when toxins build up.

Renal Failure:

- Acute kidney injury
- Chronic kidney disease

Renal and urinary function can be affected by a variety of disorders. The kidneys filter the blood making it a direct link to every other organ system.

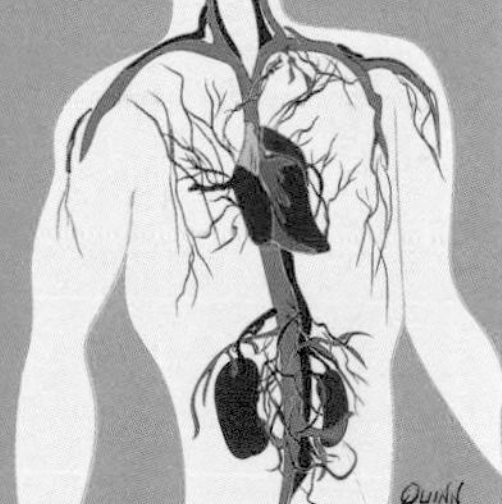

What You Need to Know

Alterations in Renal and Urinary Functions

SIGNIFICANCE OF RENAL AND URINARY FUNCTIONS

The most common problem in the urinary system is *urinary tract infection* (UTI). Any problem in the nephron can ultimately affect the body, because the kidneys filter the blood and regulate fluid, electrolyte, acid-base, and red blood cell (RBC) volume.

URINARY TRACT INFECTIONS

Cystitis—bladder is inflamed; the usual organism is *Escherichia coli.*

Pyelonephritis—renal pelvis and interstitial tissue of the kidney are inflamed.

OBSTRUCTIONS

Renal calculi—stones along the urinary tract

Neurogenic bladder—lack of bladder control due to neurologic dysfunction (brain, spinal cord, or nerve condition). Individual has no sensation of need to urinate

Structural abnormalities—birth defects or other constrictions that narrow or block the urethra

Benign prostatic hyperplasia (BPH)—prostate gland is enlarged and obstructs the flow of urine

Tumors—cancer arising from the kidneys; most often malignant (renal cell carcinoma—adenocarcinoma)

GLOMERULAR DISORDERS

Glomerulonephritis—is an autoimmune inflammatory process in the glomerulus characterized by an antigen–antibody response often to group A beta streptococcus.

Nephrotic syndrome—occurs as a result of underlying renal disease (e.g., chronic glomerulonephritis) and is characterized by large amounts of protein lost in the urine.

RENAL FAILURE

Acute kidney injury (AKI)—is characterized by a rapid loss of renal function with progressive azotemia. Causes are classified as prerenal, intrarenal, or postrenal.

Chronic kidney disease (CKD)—is progressive and the irreversible destruction of the nephrons in both kidneys characterized by stages 1 through 5—reduced renal reserve, renal insufficiency, most often leading to end-stage renal disease.

Important nursing implications

Serious/life-threatening implications

Most frequent side effects

Patient teaching

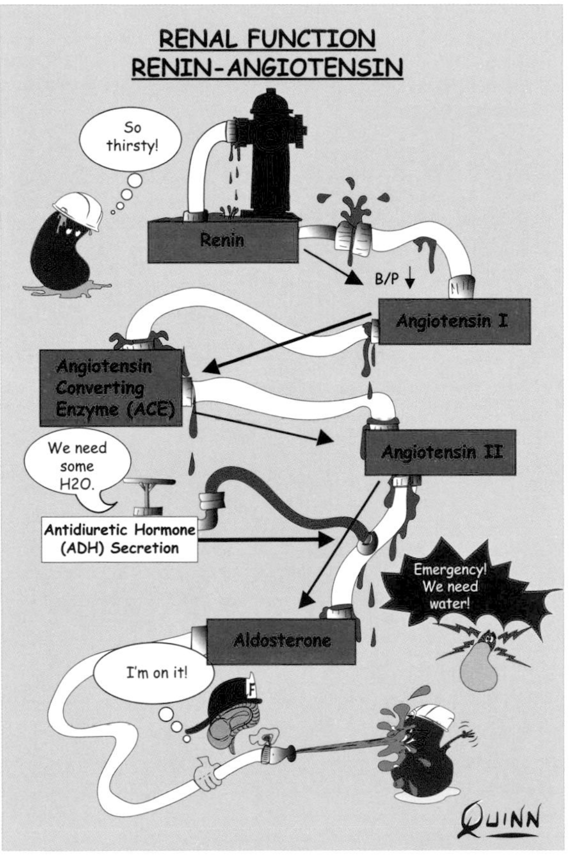
RENAL FUNCTION
RENIN-ANGIOTENSIN
So thirsty!
Renin
B/P ↓
Angiotensin I
Angiotensin Converting Enzyme (ACE)
Angiotensin II
We need some H2O.
Antidiuretic Hormone (ADH) Secretion
Emergency! We need water!
Aldosterone
I'm on it!
F
QUINN

What You Need to Know

Renal Function—Renin-Angiotensin

SIGNIFICANCE OF THE RENIN-ANGIOTENSIN SYSTEM

Renin is released in response to decreased arterial blood pressure (BP) or decreased renal blood flow or both.

MAJOR FUNCTIONS OF RENIN-ANGIOTENSIN SYSTEM

- Renin is an enzyme regulated in the juxtaglomerular apparatus of the kidney.
- Renin is released in response to decreased arterial BP, renal ischemia, extracellular fluid (ECF) depletion, increased norepinephrine, and increased urinary sodium concentration.
- Catalyzes the splitting of the plasma protein—angiotensinogen from the liver into angiotensin I.
- Enzyme from the lungs converts angiotensin I to angiotensin II via the angiotensin converting enzyme (ACE). It then simulates the release of aldosterone from the adrenal cortex, which causes sodium and water retention, resulting in increased volume of ECF.
- Angiotensin II causes an increase in peripheral vasoconstriction.
- Increased peripheral vasoconstriction along with the increase in ECF results in increased arterial BP, which ultimately inhibits the release of renin.
- Progressive release of renin may be a contributing cause to secondary hypertension.
- Because angiotensin II stimulates the secretion of the antidiuretic hormone (ADH), it also serves as an additional link between ADH and aldosterone function.

Important nursing implications | Serious/life-threatening implications

Most frequent side effects | Patient teaching

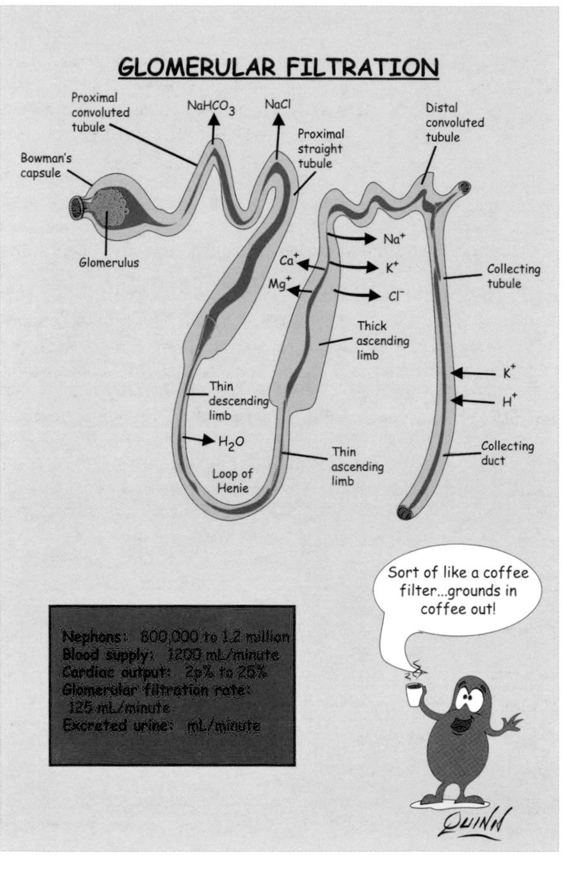
GLOMERULAR FILTRATION
Proximal convoluted tubule
$NaHCO_3$
NaCl
Proximal straight tubule
Distal convoluted tubule
Bowman's capsule
Glomerulus
Na^+
Ca^+
K^+
Mg^+
Cl^-
Collecting tubule
Thick ascending limb
K^+
H^+
Thin descending limb
H_2O
Loop of Henie
Thin ascending limb
Collecting duct
Sort of like a coffee filter...grounds in coffee out!
Nephons: 800,000 to 1.2 million
Blood supply: 1200 mL/minute
Cardiac output: 2p% to 25%
Glomerular filtration rate: 125 mL/minute
Excreted urine: mL/minute
QUINN

What You Need to Know

Glomerular Filtration

FOUR PROCESSES OF HOW THE KIDNEYS EXCRETE WASTES

1. ***Glomerular filtration***—process of ultrafiltration in which the nephron makes a filtrate of the protein-free plasma, which assists in the regulation of fluid volume, electrolyte composition, and pH levels.
2. ***Tubular reabsorption***—process in which water and solutes move from the renal tubular lumen to the peritubular capillary plasma.
3. ***Tubular secretion***—process in which substances from the peritubular capillary plasma are transferred to the renal tubular lumen.
4. ***Excretion***—process in which metabolic waste is eliminated through micturition.

GLOMERULAR FILTRATION RATE

- Approximately 125 mL/min with 99% of the filtrate is reabsorbed.
- Proximal tubule reabsorbs approximately 70% of the filtered sodium and water and 90% of the electrolytes. It reabsorbs bicarbonate, all glucose, and amino acids, and secretes hydrogen ions (H^+) and creatinine.
- Most molecules are reabsorbed by active transport. Those not reabsorbed are excreted with the urine.
- Loop of Henle reabsorbs sodium and chloride in the ascending loop. It also reabsorbs water in the descending loop, which concentrates the filtrate.
- Distal tubules use active transport to reabsorb sodium and secrete potassium and hydrogen, which assists in maintaining acid–base balance and the level of ammonia. The ADH regulates the reabsorption of water, and aldosterone regulates sodium and potassium. The distal part of the nephron regulates the excretion of H^+ and forms bicarbonate.
- Collecting duct reabsorbs water when acted on by the ADH.
- Diuretics act at different places along the nephron.

SITE OF ACTION OF DIURETICS

- Carbonic anhydrase inhibitors (Diamox)—proximal tubule
- Osmotic diuretics (mannitol)—descending loop of Henle
- Loop diuretics (Furosemide/Lasix)—ascending loop of Henle
- Thiazides (Diuril)—between end of ascending loop and beginning of distal tubule
- Potassium-sparing (spironolactone)—late distal tubule and beginning of collecting duct

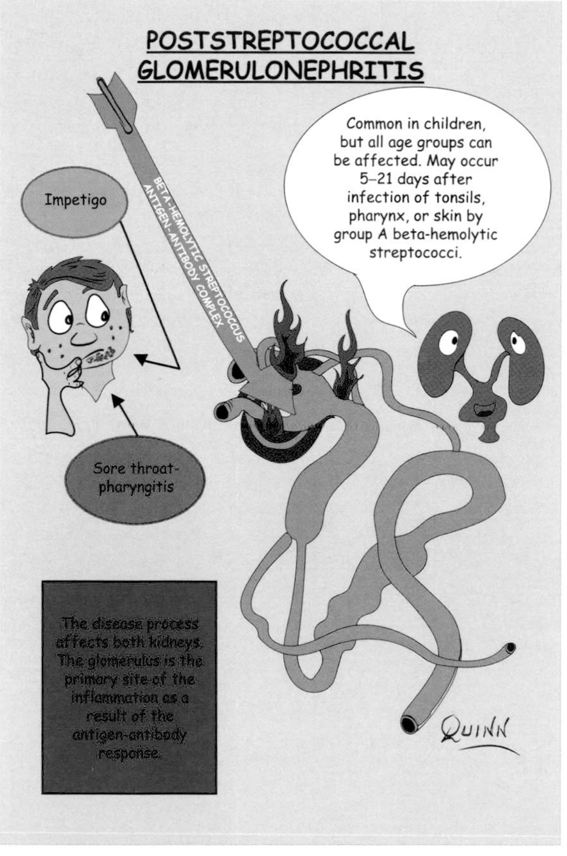
POSTSTREPTOCOCCAL GLOMERULONEPHRITIS
Common in children, but all age groups can be affected. May occur 5–21 days after infection of tonsils, pharynx, or skin by group A beta-hemolytic streptococci.
BETA-HEMOLYTIC STREPTOCOCCUS ANTIGEN-ANTIBODY COMPLEX
Impetigo
Sore throat-pharyngitis
The disease process affects both kidneys. The glomerulus is the primary site of the inflammation as a result of the antigen-antibody response.
QUINN

What You Need to Know

Glomerulonephritis

SIGNIFICANCE OF GLOMERULONEPHRITIS

Glomerulonephritis is an inflammatory process in the glomerulus caused by an antigen–antibody response related to a variety of factors but most often associated with a group A poststreptococcal infection.

TYPES OF GLOMERULONEPHRITIS

Acute Poststreptococcal Glomerulonephritis (APSGN)

- Is most common in children and young adults.
- Usually develops within 5–21 days after a streptococcal infection of the pharynx or skin.
- Antibodies are produced as a result of the streptococcal infection, leading to antigen–antibody complexes that deposit in the glomerulus, which activate complementary and inflammatory processes.

Signs and Symptoms

- Dark, reddish-brown urine
- Edema especially in face, around eyes, hands, and feet
- Oliguria, hematuria, proteinuria
- Fatigue due to low iron levels (anemia)
- Hypertension

Treatment

- Focus on limiting salt and water intake and managing blood pressure.
- Diuretic may be prescribed to increase urination.
- Administer antibiotics if streptococcal infection is still active. Educate patient on the importance of taking the antibiotic as prescribed for the full duration to prevent recurrence of problem.
- The majority of patients completely recover.
- Corticosteroids are sometimes used.

Chronic Glomerulonephritis

- End-stage glomerular inflammatory disease progresses to chronic kidney disease.

Signs and Symptoms

- Signs and symptoms may include many years of proteinuria and hematuria before diagnosis, and slow development of uremic syndrome, along with hypertension.

Treatment

- Treatment management centers around chronic kidney disease (dialysis, transplantation).

Important nursing implications | Serious/life-threatening implications
Most frequent side effects | Patient teaching

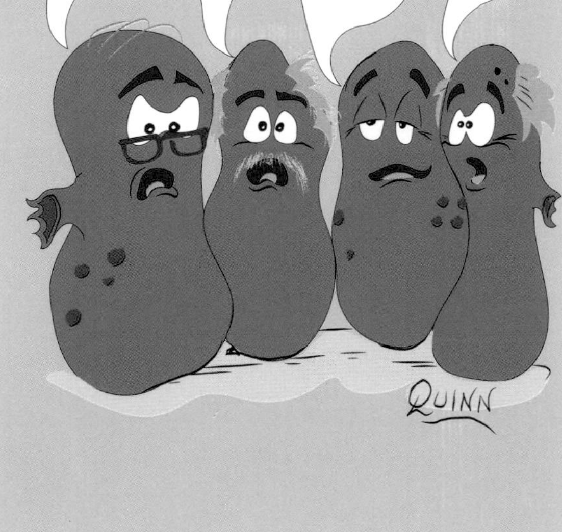
AGING AND RENAL FUNCTION
The older I get, the harder I have to work to compensate for my hypertrophy.
It's all decreasing: our nephrons, our renal flow, and our glomerular filtration rate.
I'm over 70 years old, and I have lost almost half of my glomerular function. I'm just not able to keep up with my pH and fluid loads.
My glomeruli capillaries atrophy, cutting down on my branch vessel circulation.
QUINN

What You Need to Know

Aging and Renal Function

SIGNIFICANCE OF AGING AND RENAL FUNCTION

As the body ages, there is a decline in the number of nephrons. By age 70, a 30%–50% decrease of nephrons has occurred. Most older patients are able to maintain body fluid homeostasis, despite this loss of renal function. Blood flow to the kidney decreases by approximately 10% per decade as blood vessels thicken, which causes nephrons to be more vulnerable to damage during acute episodes of hypotension or hypertension.

PHYSIOLOGIC CHANGES

- Decreases occur in both the renal blood flow and the glomerular filtration rate. The ability to conserve sodium, to dilute or concentrate urine, and to excrete an acid load also decreases. These changes can affect drug excretion because of the decreased ability to concentrate urine.
- Urinary creatinine clearance decreases and the blood urea nitrogen (BUN) level increases.
- With decreased estrogen levels in women, bladder and urethral tissues become less elastic, thin, and less vascular.
- Older women are prone to develop urethral irritation, urethral and bladder infections, overactive bladder, and urinary incontinence.
- With an enlargement of the prostate in men, urinary patterns are characterized by hesitancy, retention, slow stream, and bladder infections.
- Decline in renal function is more rapid in patients with diabetes, hypertension, or heart failure.

Important nursing implications	Serious/life-threatening implications
Most frequent side effects	Patient teaching

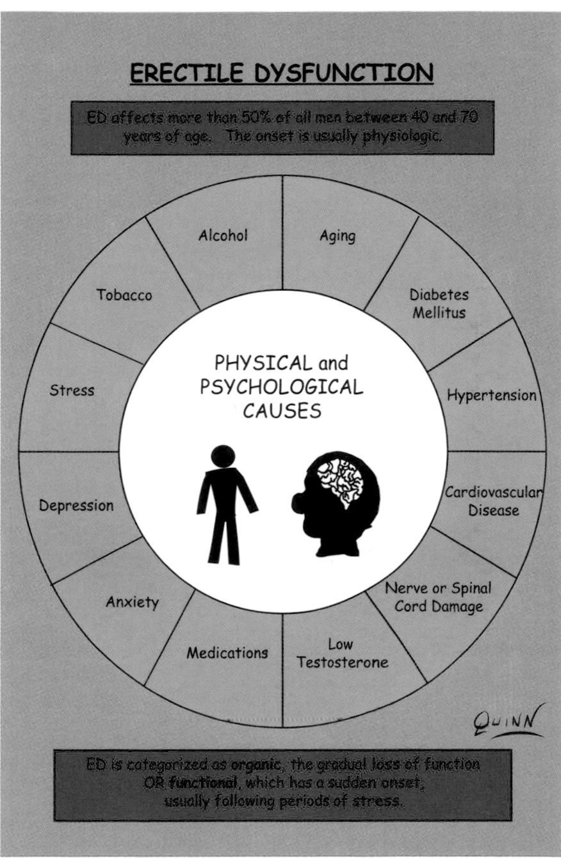
ERECTILE DYSFUNCTION
ED affects more than 50% of all men between 40 and 70 years of age. The onset is usually physiologic.
Alcohol
Aging
Tobacco
Diabetes Mellitus
PHYSICAL and PSYCHOLOGICAL CAUSES
Stress
Hypertension
Depression
Cardiovascular Disease
Anxiety
Nerve or Spinal Cord Damage
Medications
Low Testosterone
QUINN
ED is categorized as organic, the gradual loss of function OR functional, which has a sudden onset, usually following periods of stress.

What You Need to Know

Erectile Dysfunction

Erectile dysfunction (ED), also known as impotence, is the inability to achieve or maintain an erection for sexual intercourse. ED affects more than 50% of all men between 40 and 70 years of age. ED is categorized as either *organic* (gradual) or *functional* (sudden).

TYPES OF ED

Organic ED

- Is characterized by the gradual deterioration of function.
- Symptoms include a diminished firmness and a decrease in the frequency of erection.
- Causes include the following:
  - Inflammation of the prostate, urethra, or seminal vesicles
  - Pelvic and lumbosacral injuries
  - Neurologic conditions (Parkinson disease, multiple sclerosis)
  - Diabetes, thyroid problems
  - Smoking, alcohol consumption
  - Antihypertensive medications

Functional ED

- Is characterized by a sudden loss of function, usually following a period of high stress.
- Men usually have normal nocturnal (nighttime) and morning erections.

TREATMENT

- Oral drug therapy includes Viagra, Cialis, or Levitra.
- Vacuum device—device fits over the penis, and blood is drawn into the penis using a pump. A rubber ring (tension band) is placed at the base of penis to maintain the erection.
- Intracorporal injections—vasodilating drugs injected directly into the penis.
- Intraurethral applications—urethral suppository
- Penile implants—prosthesis is used when other modalities fail and involves a surgical procedure.

NURSING MANAGEMENT

- Educate the individual in understanding the implications of the medications or devices used to treat ED and assist in obtaining counseling.

- Educate the individual about how ED medications can potentiate the hypotensive effects of nitrates and should not be taken at the same time.
- Abstain from alcohol if taking ED medications.

Important nursing implications | Serious/life-threatening implications
Most frequent side effects | Patient teaching

BENIGN PROSTATIC HYPERTROPHY (BPH)

BPH is nonmalignant growth or hyperplasia of prostate tissue starting around age 40 years and affecting 80% of men over age 70 years.

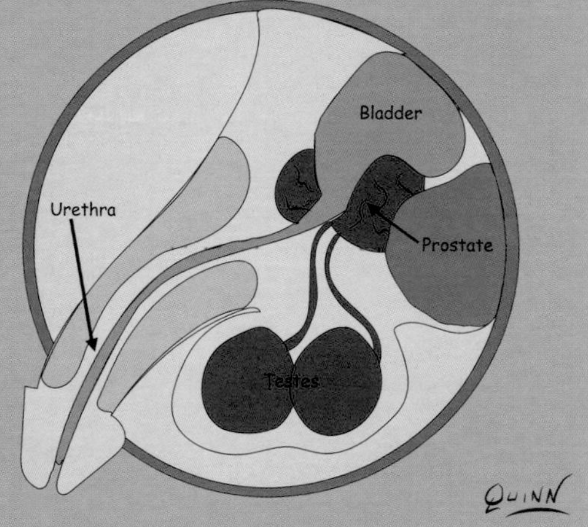

Common Symptoms:

- Frequency
- Urgency
- Dysuria
- Bladder Pain
- Nocturia
- Incontinence

Obstructive Symptoms:

- Decrease in stream and force
- Hesitation in urination
- Postvoid dribbling
- Eventual acute urinary retention is an indication for surgical intervention

What You Need to Know

Benign Prostatic Hypertrophy

Benign prostatic hypertrophy (BPH), or hyperplasia, is an enlargement of prostate gland tissue. High levels of dihydrotestosterone (DHT), a testosterone derivative, may accumulate in the prostrate and increase cell growth. Enlargement of the gland causes bladder outlet obstruction, which leads to the following signs and symptoms.

SIGNS AND SYMPTOMS

- Hypertrophy of the detrusor (bladder muscle)—because of thickening, the prostate cannot effectively contract.
- Urinary frequency, hesitancy particularly on initiation of voiding, nocturia, and/or hematuria.
- Diminished force of urinary stream.
- Increased residual urine (postvoid) leads to overflow urinary incontinence (i.e., dribbling).
- Urinary retention, which may become acute. Chronic urinary retention can lead to a backup of urine, resulting in bladder distention, hydroureter, and hydronephrosis.

DIAGNOSTIC FINDINGS

- Abnormal digital rectal examination
- Elevated prostate-specific antigen (PSA) serum blood test
- Abnormal cystoscopy and bladder scan or transrectal and/or transabdominal ultrasound
- Positive urinalysis with culture and sensitivity for bacteria identification

TREATMENT

Medical

- Generic finasteride (Proscar) and alpha-adrenergic blockers shrink prostatic tissue.
- Radiation, hormonal therapy, and chemotherapy to treat malignancy.

Surgical:

Size of the prostate and the patient's general health dictate the type of surgery.

- Transurethral resection of the prostate (TURP): Prostatic tissue is removed via a resectoscope, which is passed through the urethra.

- Transurethral incision of the prostate (TUIP): Makes transurethral slits or incisions into prostate to relieve obstruction. Procedure is effective with minimally enlarged prostate (BPH).
- Prostatectomy: Prostate is removed via a suprapubic, retropubic, or perineal approach and may be performed by incision or laparoscopically. It is most often the procedure of choice for the removal of malignancy.
- Transurethral microwave therapy (TUMT) and transurethral needle ablation (TUNA): Microwave energy is delivered directly to the prostate. Heat causes necrosis of tissue. Both procedures are performed on an outpatient basis.
- Internal radiation therapy (brachytherapy): Involves the placement of tiny radioactive "seeds" into the prostate for the treatment of cancer.
- Hormone therapy (antiandrogen medications [Lupron]): Deprives the cancer cells of testosterone, which may help slow the growth of prostatic cancer.
- Cryotherapy (cryoablation): Liquid nitrogen is applied to the prostate via a transrectal ultrasound probe. Dead cells are absorbed by the body.

Important nursing implications	Serious/life-threatening implications
Most frequent side effects	Patient teaching

MENSTRUAL ALTERATIONS

Dysmenorrhea
(Painful menstruation)

Amenorrhea
(Absence of menstruation)

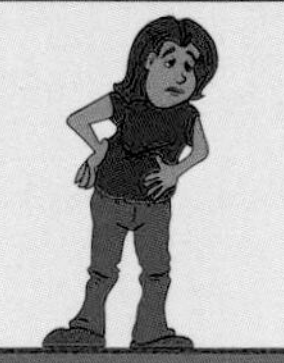

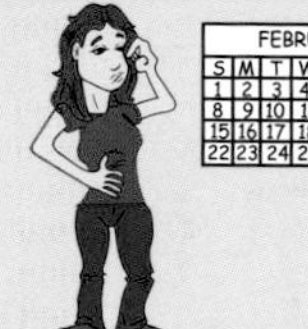

Discomfort usually starts within 12–24 hours before the onset of menses.

Primary: No menarche by age 16 or age 14 years with development of secondary characteristics.
Secondary: Cessation of menses after initiation, triggered by malnutrition, pregnancy, lactation, and menopause.

Hypermenorrhea
(Abnormal menstruation)

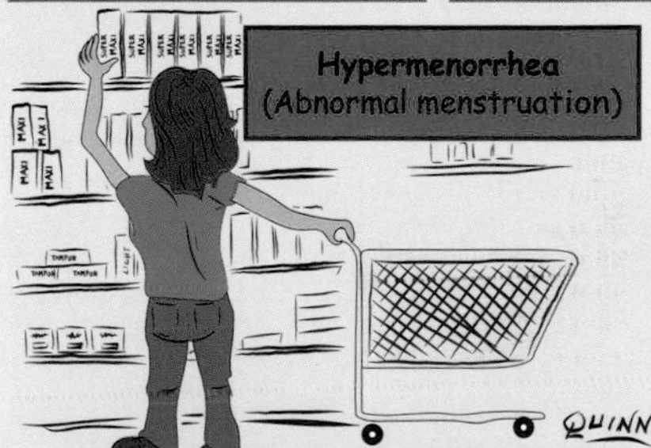

Menorrhagia: Increased amount and duration of flow
Metrorrhagia: Irregular bleeding episodes between menstrual cycles

What You Need to Know

Menstrual Alterations

DYSMENORRHEA

- Starts within 12 and 24 hours before the onset of menses.
- Pain is the most severe on the first day of menses and rarely lasts more than 2 days.
- Pain may radiate into the groin and be accompanied by backache, anorexia, vomiting, diarrhea, syncope, and headache.

TYPES

- *Primary*— painful menstruation is associated with the release of prostaglandins in the ovulatory cycle.
- *Secondary*— painful menstruation related to pelvic disease, such as endometriosis, chronic pelvic inflammatory disease (PID), and uterine fibroids.

AMENORRHEA

- Menses is lacking.
- Infertility, vasomotor flushes, vaginal atrophy, acne, osteopenia, and hirsutism may also be present and are associated with the underlying cause of the amenorrhea.

TYPES

- *Primary*—menarche fails by the age of 16 years or by the age of 14 years with the development of secondary sex characteristics.
- *Secondary*—cessation of menses after initial onset. Associated with dramatic weight loss (triggered by malnutrition or excessive exercise), or occurs during pregnancy, lactation, and menopause.

HYPERMENORRHEA

- Menstrual bleeding is abnormal. Hypermenorrhea may be a sign of an abnormal condition.

TYPES

- *Menorrhea*—prolonged menstrual flow
- *Menorrhagia*—increased amount and duration of flow

- *Metrorrhagia*—irregular bleeding between periods (think of the ***t*** in me***t***rorrhagia and be***t***ween to help remember the different types of hypermenorrhea).

Important nursing implications
Serious/life-threatening implications
Most frequent side effects
Patient teaching

DISORDERS OF THE PENIS AND SCROTUM

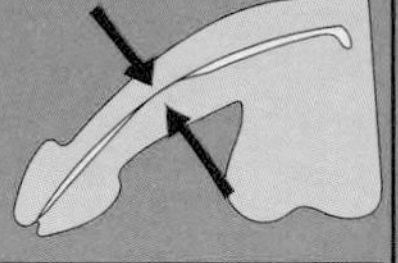

Urethral strictures...fibrotic scar tissue blocking the release of urine. Need to remove blockage before damage, abscess, or infection occur.

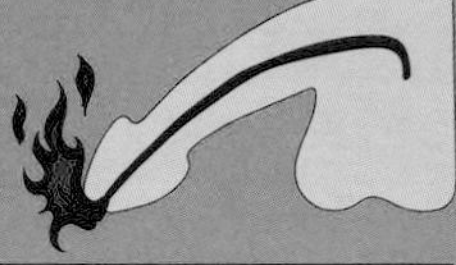

Urethritis...an inflammation of the urethra, can be caused from a sexually transmitted disease. Symptoms include burning with urination, penile itching, and discharge.

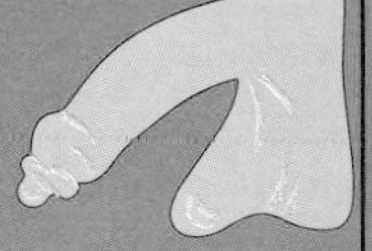

Phimosis...the foreskin cannot be retracted back over the glans penis.

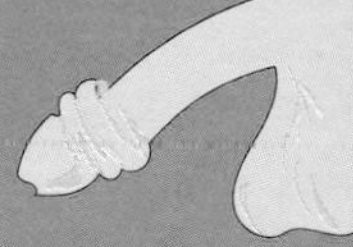

Paraphimosis...the foreskin is retracted and cannot be moved forward to cover the glans penis causing edema and decreasing circulation. This is a medical emergency.

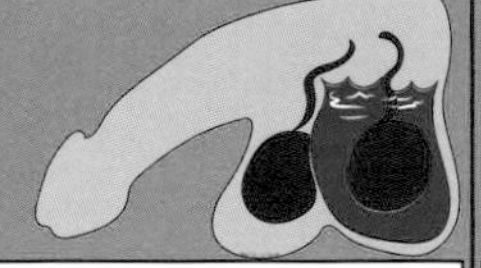

Hydrocele...swelling in the scrotum from fluid collection surrounding a testicle. More common in newborns, but can occur after injury to the area in older males.

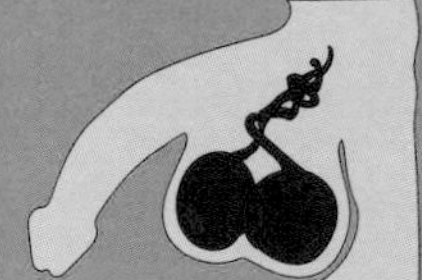

Testicular torsion...the twisting of spermatic cord causing blood flow interruption to the scrotum causing sudden, severe pain and swelling. Requires emergency care.

What You Need to Know

Disorders of the Penis and Scrotum

DISORDERS OF THE PENIS

Urethral Strictures

- Lumen of the urethra is narrowed.
- Trauma surgery or congenital defect is the cause, as well as sexually transmitted infections (STIs) (e.g., chlamydia).
- Signs and symptoms include a diminished force of urinary stream, spraying, or split urinary stream, feelings of incomplete bladder emptying, frequency, nocturia, dysuria, and discharge.

Urethritis

- Inflammation of the urethra.
- Most often caused by STIs (e.g., gonorrhea), but can also be from a bacterial or viral infection.
- Signs and symptoms include discharge (purulent—gonococcal infection; nonpurulent—nongonococcal infection), dysuria, and frequent urination.

Phimosis and Paraphimosis

- Foreskin is too tight to move easily over the glans penis.
- Phimosis—foreskin cannot be retracted back over the glans penis.
- Paraphimosis—foreskin is retracted and cannot be moved forward to cover the glans penis. This is a medical emergency.
- Can occur at any age and is associated with poor hygiene and infection.
- Signs and symptoms include edema, erythema, tenderness, and purulent discharge.

DISORDERS OF THE SCROTUM

Hydrocele

- Fluid collects in the tunica vaginalis.
- Imbalance between secreting and absorptive capacities of scrotal tissues is usually the cause.
- Compression of testicular blood supply may lead to atrophy.

Torsion of the Testes

- Rotation of a testis can twist blood vessels in the spermatic cord causing blood flow interruption. Requires emergent medical care.

- Signs and symptoms include testicular pain and a swelling that may spontaneously occur after physical exertion or trauma, as well as vascular engorgement and ischemia, along with an absent cremasteric reflex.

Important nursing implications
Serious/life-threatening implications
Most frequent side effects
Patient teaching

PUBERTY

Precocious Puberty (Early)

I'm 7 years old and my breasts are growing, but my bones have stopped. I'm going to be short.
Isosexual

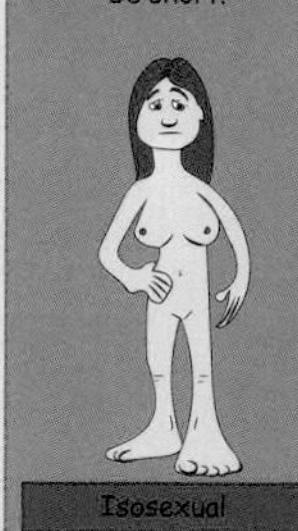

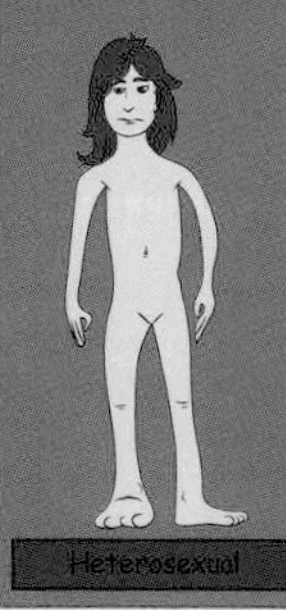

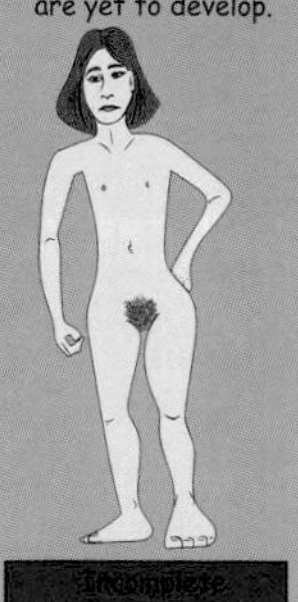

Delayed Puberty

I'm 16 years old. Where are my breasts? When will I have my first period?

95% of delayed puberty occurs in young women with normal hypothalmic-pituitary-ovarian axis...but 5% are caused by a disruption of the hypothalmic-pituitary-gonadal axis...either acquired congenitally or through systemic disease.

QUINN

What You Need to Know

Puberty

SIGNIFICANCE OF PUBERTY

Puberty is the process of sexual maturation. It is marked by the development of secondary sex characteristics, rapid body growth, and the ability to reproduce.

DELAYED PUBERTY

- Secondary sex characteristics have not appeared by age 13 years in girls (breast development) or age 14 years in boys (testicular development).
- Is related to chronic disease (renal failure, lung disease, cystic fibrosis) or is a result of corticosteroid use in adolescents with asthma.

Treatment

- Trial of exogenous sex hormones promotes positive self-image and as a diagnostic measure for irreversible hypogonadotropism.

PRECOCIOUS PUBERTY

Sexual maturation occurs before age 6 in black girls or age 7 in white girls and before age 9 in boys. Precocious puberty occurs in three forms.

Isosexual

- Is GnRH-dependent and occurs when the hypothalamic-pituitary-gonadal axis is working normally but prematurely.

Heterosexual

- Virilization of a girl and feminization of a boy causes the child to develop some secondary sex characteristics of the opposite sex.
- Condition present at birth and is rare in older children.

Incomplete

- Secondary sex characteristics are only partially developed.
- Does not progress to complete puberty (ovulation, menstruation).
- Majority of children with precocious puberty are obese.

Treatment

- Medication—usually consists of GnRH agonists, which induce reversible, selective suppression of the pituitary-gonadal axis.

Important nursing implications	Serious/life-threatening implications
Most frequent side effects	Patient teaching

MENSTRUAL CYCLE

The menstrual cycle is the monthly hormonal cycle a female's body goes through to prepare for pregnancy.

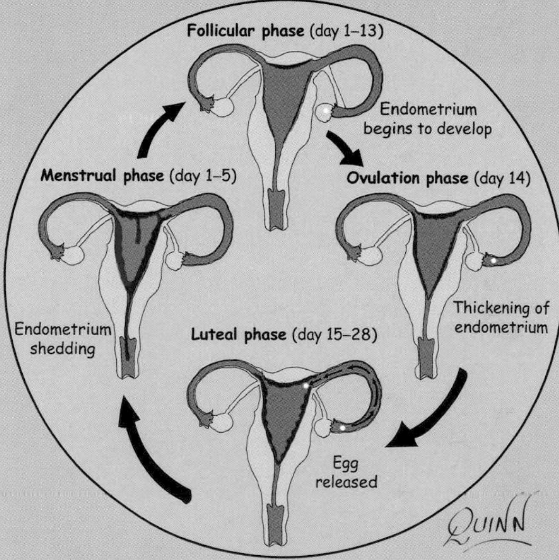

Hormone levels fluctuate throughout the menstrual cycle, which can cause mood changes, asthma, irritable bowel disease, and bladder pain syndrome.

What You Need to Know

Menstrual Cycle

PHASES OF MENSTRUAL CYCLE

Proliferative or Follicular

- Involves the maturation of an ovarian follicle and the proliferation of the endometrium.
- Anterior pituitary gland secretes a follicle-stimulating hormone (FSH), which promotes follicle development.
- Granulosa cells of the follicle secrete estrogen, which causes endometrial cells to proliferate. This proliferation induces a luteotropic hormone (LH) surge, which causes progesterone production in the ovary.
- When the follicle is mature, the endometrial lining is restored, fully proliferated, and able to support an embryo.

Secretory or Luteal

- Involves ovulation. Ovarian follicle transforms into a corpus luteum.
- LH from the anterior pituitary gland is responsible for simulating the corpus luteum to secrete progesterone, which initiates the secretory phase.
- Glands and blood vessels begin to coil in the endometrium and secrete a thin, glycogen-containing fluid, as well as dilate the glandular ducts.
- If conception occurs, then the endometrium is ready. If conception does not occur, then the corpus luteum degenerates and stops producing progesterone and estrogen.
- Blood vessels contract and tissue sloughs away (without conception). The process results in menses and the initiation of the menstrual phase.

Menstrual or Ischemic

- Menstrual phase involves menstruation (menses) during which the functional layer of the endometrium disintegrates and is sloughed off via vaginal bleeding.
- Begins on the first day of menses and lasts 3–7 days. The amount of blood loss is normally between 30 and 80 mL with the majority of blood loss occurring during the first 3 days.
- Estrogen levels are low; minute amounts of progesterone are secreted.
- Menstrual discharge consists of blood, mucus, and desquamated endometrial tissue and should not clot under normal circumstances.

Important nursing implications | Serious/life-threatening implications
Most frequent side effects | Patient teaching

INFERTILITY

It's been over a year without any protection. Why can't we conceive a child?
Infertility affects approximately 15% of all couples. Treatment is aimed at correcting the underlying cause.
QUINN

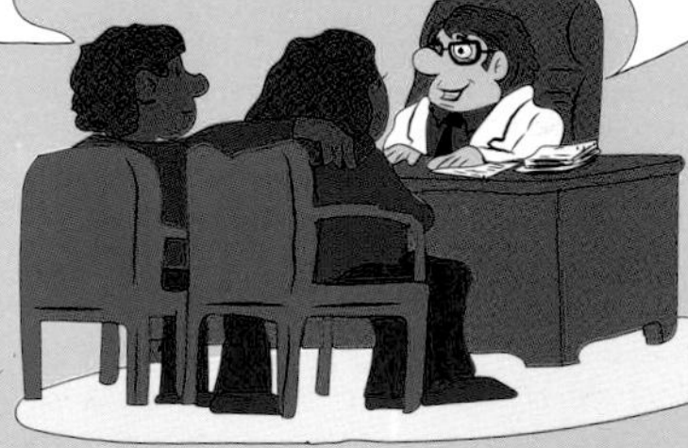

Female Problems

- Malfunctions in the fallopian tubes and ovaries, which could be genetic or be caused by adhesions from infections that might block sperm
- Inadequate equality or quantity of reproductive hormones

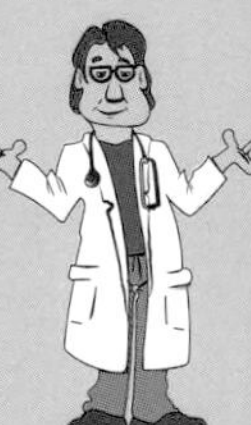

Male Problems

- Compromised quality of sperm
  - Decreased number of viable sperm
  - Poor structure
  - Decreased mobility
- Obstructions along the reproductive tract

It is important to provide early reproduction education to couples wanting to conceive. Early prevention, detection, and treatment of sexually transmitted diseases are the best approaches to healthy reproductive function and fertility.

What You Need to Know

Infertility

SIGNIFICANCE OF INFERTILITY

Infertility is the inability to achieve a pregnancy after at least 1 year of regular intercourse. Infertility affects about 15% of all couples.

CAUSES OF INFERTILITY

Women

- Malfunction in the fallopian tubes and/or ovaries, which may be genetic
- Anovulation, tubal obstruction or dysfunction (endometriosis or damage from PID), and uterine or cervical factors
- Risk factors include tobacco and illicit drug use, infection of the reproductive tract, and increasing age

Men

- Compromised quality of sperm or obstruction along reproductive tract
- Decreased number of viable sperm, poor sperm structure, or decreased sperm motility

DIAGNOSTIC STUDIES

- Ovulatory studies—determination of basal body temperature; drop in temperature as ovulation approaches
- Tubal patency studies—x-ray studies of the uterus and tubes with a radiopaque dye injected through the cervix
- Postcoital studies—examination of the cervical mucus to reveal whether it undergoes favorable changes at ovulation
- Sperm counts/semen analysis—assessment of number and mobility of sperm

TREATMENT

- Management of infertility depends on the cause.
- Early prevention, detection, and treatment of STIs.
- If infertility is related to ovarian problems, then supplemental hormone therapy is usually indicated.
- If related to chronic cervicitis and inadequate estrogenic stimulation, then antibiotics for the cervicitis and estrogen administration may be indicated.
- Other treatment includes intrauterine insemination with partner or donor sperm or, if insemination is ineffective, possible in vitro fertilization.

MENOPAUSE

Complications of Menopause
- Increased incidence of osteoporosis
- Increased risk for cardiovascular disease

Perimenopause
- Irregular bleeding
- Hot flashes
- Erratic hormone fluctuation
- Decreased estrogen
- Breast tenderness
- Mood changes

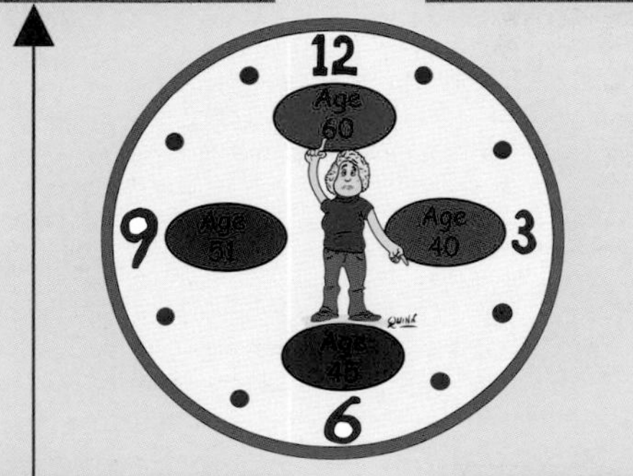

Menopause
- Menopause is the complete cessation of menstruation after 12 months.
- Decreased ovarian function starts before the age of 40 years

Menopause Transition
- Vasomotor symptoms
- Stress and urge incontinence
- Dyspareunia
- Slowed metabolism
- Vaginal dryness
- Atrophy of vaginal tissue

Menopause happens to all women, generally starting between ages 40 and 60 years, with an average age of 51 years.

What You Need to Know

Menopause

SIGNIFICANCE OF MENOPAUSE

Perimenopause is a term used to describe the stages of a woman's life that begins with the first sign of change in the menstrual cycle and ends after menses ceases. *Menopause* is the complete cessation of menses after 12 months. *Postmenopause* refers to the time after menopause.

SIGNS AND SYMPTOMS

Perimenopause

- Irregular vaginal bleeding, vasomotor instability (hot flashes and night sweats), atrophy of the genitourinary tissue, hormone fluctuation, stress and urge incontinence
- Breast tenderness, mood changes

Post-Menopause

- Cessation of menses, occasional vasomotor symptoms
- Continued atrophy of genitourinary tissue with diminished support
- Stress and urge incontinence, osteoporosis

Other Symptoms of Estrogen Deficiency

- Increased risk for cardiovascular disease
- Decreased high-density lipoproteins (HDL); increased low-density lipoproteins (LDL); diminished collagen content of skin; breast tissue changes
- Increased fracture rate—especially vertebral bodies, humerus, distal radius, upper femur
- Emotional lability, change in sleep pattern, decreased rapid eye movement (REM) sleep

TREATMENT

- Hormone replacement therapy (HRT)—should be thoroughly discussed with the patient. The patient's choice is based on risk factors. History of breast cancer is generally a contraindication for HRT.

- Herbs and supplemental therapies—phytoestrogens (soy, tofu, chick peas, sunflower seeds), black cohosh, dang quai.
  - Encourage patient to consult with healthcare provider about taking phytoestrogens and other herbal products.

Important nursing implications

Serious/life-threatening implications

Most frequent side effects

Patient teaching

SEXUALLY TRANSMITTED INFECTIONS

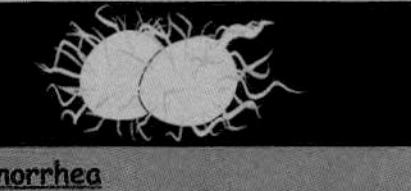

Gonorrhea
(Neisseria gonorrhoeae)
Contact with epithelial surfaces during oral, anal, or genital intercourse. Causes urethritis, dysuria, and purulent drainage from the urethra.

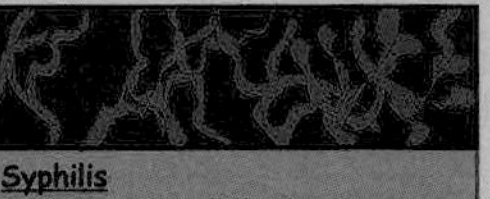

Syphilis
(Treponema pallidum)
Contact with moist mucosal or cutaneous lesions and minor abrasions during sexual intercourse. Becomes systemic.

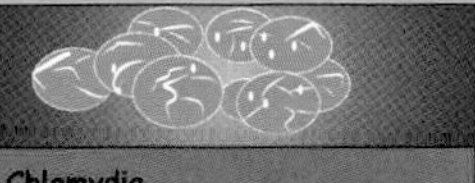

Chlamydia
(Chlamydia trachomatis)
Bacterial STI affecting men and women. Causes urethritis in men, damages the woman's reproductive system, and can cause ectopic pregnancy.

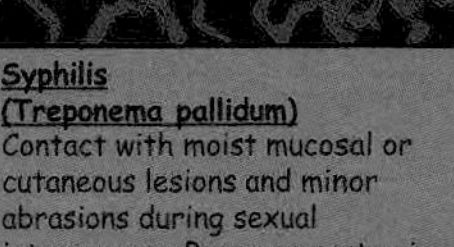

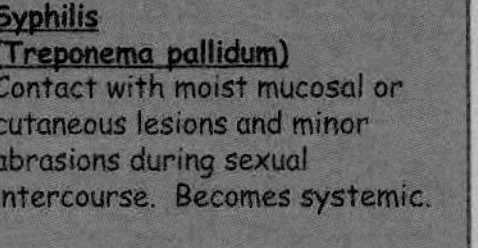

Genital Herpes—Viral
Contracted via intimate contact with a person who is shedding the virus (most likely at a time when the carrier is a symptomatic).

Quinn

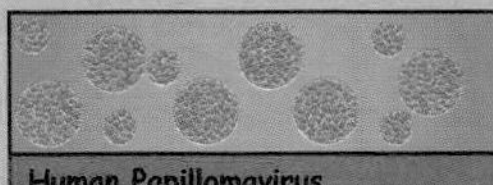

Human Papillomavirus
(Condyloma acuminata)
The most common STI. Transmitted via sexual contact. Persons infected can be asymptomatic but transmit it to others. HPV is linked to cancer.

Trichomoniasis
(Trichomonas vaginalis)
Caused by a protozoan parasite. Symptoms are more common in women and include foul smelling discharge, itching, and dysuria.

What You Need to Know

Sexually Transmitted Infections

GONORRHEA

- Is caused by the bacteria, *Neisseria gonorrhoeae,* and is the most common sexually transmitted disease (STD).
- Transmission is through direct contact with exudate via sexual contact or to the neonate during passage through the birth canal.
- Signs and symptoms include dysuria, abnormal vaginal or penis discharge, abdomen pain, or may be asymptomatic.

SYPHILIS

- Is caused by the spirochete, *Treponema pallidum.*
- Transmission is through direct contact with the primary chancre lesion or body secretions (saliva, blood, vaginal discharge, semen) and is transmitted transplacentally to the fetus.
- Signs and symptoms include chancre, painless ulcers, body rash, fatigue, swollen glands.

CHLAMYDIA INFECTION

- Nongonococcal urethritis is caused by *Chlamydia trachomatis*.
- Transmission is through direct sexual contact.
- Signs and symptoms include dysuria, dyspareunia, and abnormal vaginal or penile discharge.

HERPES GENITALIS (TYPE II)

- Is caused by type II herpes virus hominis (HVH).
- Transmission is through direct contact with the vesicles. Increased documentation indicates asymptomatic shedding and transmission of the virus.
- Signs and symptoms include painful vesicles surrounded by an erythematous area, which progress to shallow ulcers, pustules, and crusts. Spontaneous healing occurs in approximately 2–4 weeks during the initial infection.

CONDYLOMATA ACUMINATA (GENITAL WARTS)

- Is caused by the human papilloma virus (HPV).
- Transmitted through direct sexual contact. HPV is continually shed, and reinfection is common.
- Signs and symptoms are characterized by a cluster of warts.

TRICHOMONIASIS

- Is caused by the protozoan parasite *Trichomonas vaginalis.*
- Transmission through sexual intercourse.
- Signs and symptoms include itching, burning, redness, and soreness of genitals.

Important nursing implications | Serious/life-threatening implications

Most frequent side effects | Patient teaching

PRIMARY SKIN LESIONS

Macule

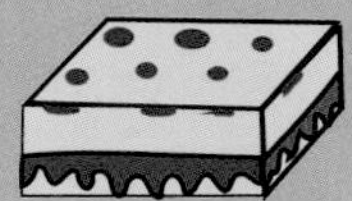

- Flat, circumscribed, discolored area
- Less than 1 cm in diameter
- Example: Freckles

Pustule

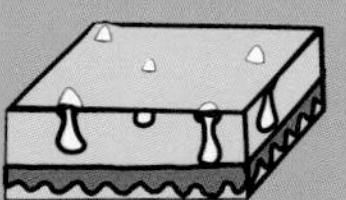

- Elevated, superficial lesion, filled with purulent fluid (pus); inflammatory
- Variable size
- Example: Acne

Papule

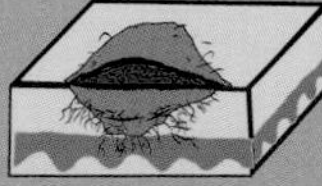

- Elevated, firm, circumscribed area
- Less than 1 cm in diameter
- Example: Wart (verruca)

Wheal

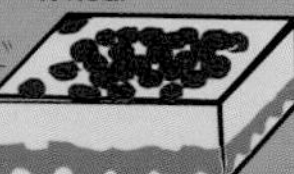

- Elevated, irregular-shaped, transient area of cutaneous edema
- Variable diameter
- Example: Allergic reaction

Vesicle

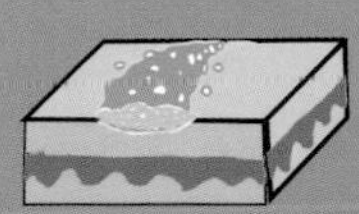

- Elevated, circumscribed, superficial lesion, filled with serous fluid
- Less than 1 cm
- Example: Herpes zoster (shingles)

Plaque

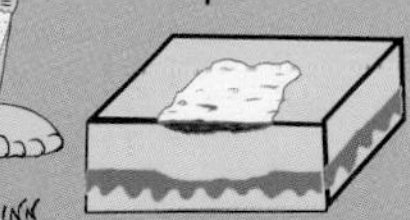

Quinn

- Elevated, firm, and rough lesion with flat top surface
- Greater than 1 cm in diameter
- Example: Psoriasis

What You Need to Know

Primary Skin Lesions

SIGNIFICANCE OF PRIMARY SKIN LESIONS

Primary lesions develop on previously unaltered skin and are considered early skin changes that have not yet undergone natural evolution or changes caused by manipulation.

TYPES OF LESIONS

Macule

- Macule lesions are flat, variably shaped, discolored, and small (<1 cm).
- Examples include freckles, flat moles, tattoos, port-wine stains, and rashes of rickettsial infections, rubella, measles, and some allergic drug eruptions.

Papule

- Papule lesions are solid, elevated, and usually <1 cm
- Examples include warts and some elevated nevi (moles).

Plaque

- Elevated, rough, plateau like lesions that measure >1 cm
- Examples include psoriasis, syphilitic chancre, lichen planus, and seborrheic and actinic keratoses.

Vesicle

- Circumscribed, elevated lesions contain serous fluid and measure <1 cm
- If lesion measures >1 cm, then it is called a *bulla* (blister).
- Vesicles or bullae are caused by primary irritants, allergic contact dermatitis, physical trauma, sunburn, insect bites, or viral infections (herpes simplex, varicella, herpes zoster).

Wheals (Hives)

- Transient, elevated, irregular-shaped areas of cutaneous edema that are solid with variable diameters.
- Common causative factor includes allergic reactions (e.g., drug eruptions; insect stings or bites; sensitivity to cold, heat, pressure, or sunlight)

Pustule

- Superficial and an elevated lesion that contains pus.
- May be the result of infection or seropurulent evolution of vesicles or bullae.
- Some causes are impetigo, acne, folliculitis, furuncles, and carbuncles.

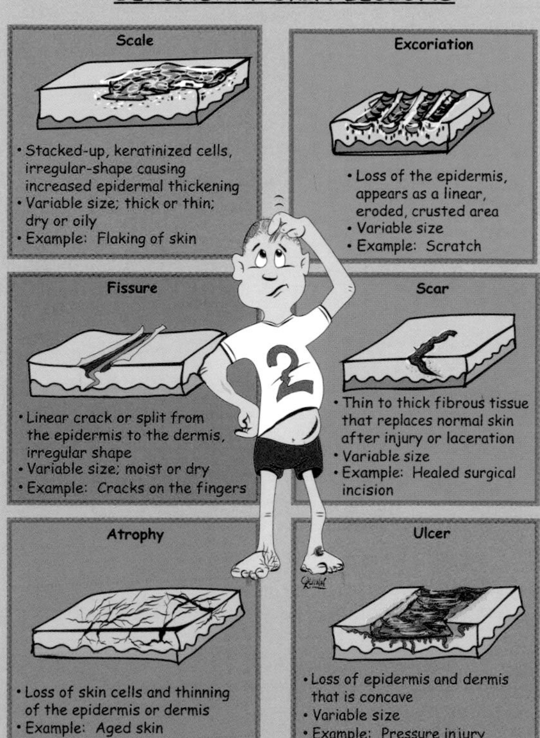
SECONDARY SKIN LESIONS
Scale
• Stacked-up, keratinized cells, irregular-shape causing increased epidermal thickening
• Variable size; thick or thin; dry or oily
• Example: Flaking of skin
Excoriation
• Loss of the epidermis, appears as a linear, eroded, crusted area
• Variable size
• Example: Scratch
Fissure
• Linear crack or split from the epidermis to the dermis, irregular shape
• Variable size; moist or dry
• Example: Cracks on the fingers
Scar
• Thin to thick fibrous tissue that replaces normal skin after injury or laceration
• Variable size
• Example: Healed surgical incision
Atrophy
• Loss of skin cells and thinning of the epidermis or dermis
• Example: Aged skin
Ulcer
• Loss of epidermis and dermis that is concave
• Variable size
• Example: Pressure injury
2

What You Need to Know

Secondary Skin Lesions

SIGNIFICANCE OF SECONDARY SKIN LESIONS

Secondary skin lesions result from external factors such as scratching, trauma, infection, diseases, or changes in the way skin heals.

SCALES

- Flakes or particles of desquamated skin cells are characteristic.
- Heaped-up particles of horny epithelium develop.
- Most common scaling rashes are from psoriasis, seborrheic dermatitis, superficial fungal infections, tinea versicolor, pityriasis rosea, and chronic dermatitis of any type.

ULCER

- Focal loss of the epidermis and at least part of the dermis occur.
- Appears concave and varies in size.
- When an ulcer is the result of a physical trauma or an acute bacterial infection, the cause is usually apparent.
- Pressure on bony prominences (coccyx) may cause ulcerations if pressure is not relieved.

EXCORIATION

- Linear or hollowed-out crusted area is observed.
- Is caused by scratching, rubbing, or picking.

ATROPHY

- Loss of skin cells and thinning of the epidermis and dermis.
- Paper-thin, wrinkled skin develops with a loss of skin markings.
- Occurs in the older adult population.

SCARS

- Areas of fibrous tissue replace normal skin after the destruction of some of the dermis.
- May be caused by burns or cuts or less commonly by diseases (e.g., discoid lupus erythematosis [LE]).

FISSURE

- Linear crack or break from the epidermis to the dermis develops (e.g., athlete's foot [fungal infection] and cracks at the corner of the mouth).
- May be dry or moist.

Important nursing implications

Serious/life-threatening implications

Most frequent side effects

Patient teaching

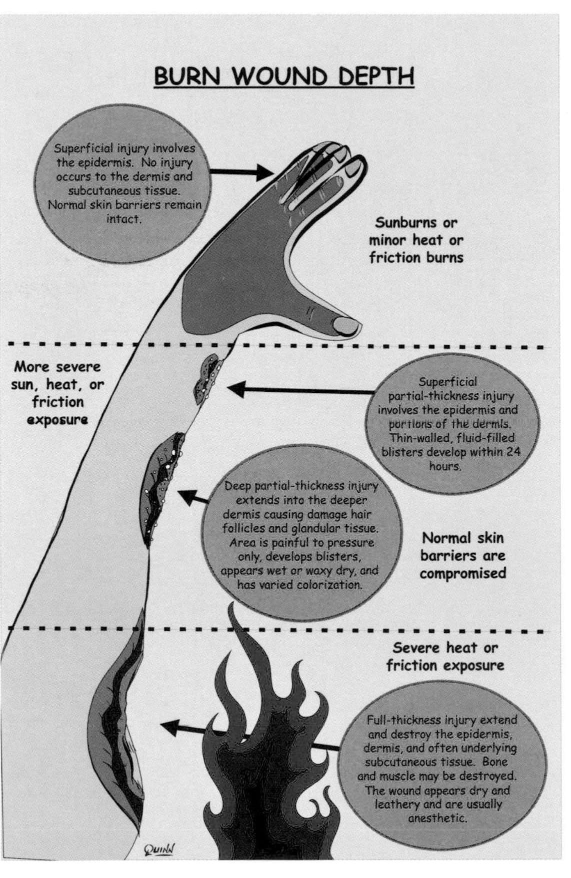
BURN WOUND DEPTH
Superficial injury involves the epidermis. No injury occurs to the dermis and subcutaneous tissue. Normal skin barriers remain intact.
Sunburns or minor heat or friction burns
More severe sun, heat, or friction exposure
Superficial partial-thickness injury involves the epidermis and portions of the dermis. Thin-walled, fluid-filled blisters develop within 24 hours.
Deep partial-thickness injury extends into the deeper dermis causing damage hair follicles and glandular tissue. Area is painful to pressure only, develops blisters, appears wet or waxy dry, and has varied colorization.
Normal skin barriers are compromised
Severe heat or friction exposure
Full-thickness injury extend and destroy the epidermis, dermis, and often underlying subcutaneous tissue. Bone and muscle may be destroyed. The wound appears dry and leathery and are usually anesthetic.
QUINN

What You Need to Know

Burn Wound Depth

BURN WOUND DEPTH

Partial Thickness

- *First-degree wound—superficial destruction (involves epidermis only)*
    - Erythema, blanching on pressure, and pain with mild swelling occurs; no initial blistering develops, but the wound may blister and peel after 24 hours.
- *Second-degree wound—destruction of epidermis and dermis*
    - Superficial partial thickness—involves *superficial dermis*. Fluid-filled blisters are red, shiny, or wet if vesicles have ruptured; severe pain is the result of nerve injury; mild-to-moderate edema develops.
- Deep partial thickness—*Involves deeper dermis*. Appears waxy-white, and often a layer of flat, dehydrated "tissue paper" lifts off in sheets; usually takes weeks to heal.

Full Thickness

- *Third-degree wound—damage of the lower layers of the dermis and underlying tissue.*
    - Blisters are rare; burn wound may be white, cherry red, or black in color with leathery or hard skin; thrombosed vessels are visible.
    - Insensitivity to pain and pressure are due to nerve tissue destruction.
    - May have involvement of muscles, tendons, and bones.
    - Removal of the damaged tissue results in a defect that must be filled with granulation tissue to heal.

TYPES OF BURN INJURIES

- Chemical injury—is the result of contact with a corrosive substance.
- Electrical injury—intense heat is generated from electrical current and causes coagulation necrosis as it flows through the body.
- Thermal injury—is the most common type of burn injury that results from flames, flash (explosion), scald, or direct contact.
- Inhalation injury—results from the inhalation of smoke and asphyxiates. The respiratory system frequently sustains two types of burn injuries:
    - Smoke inhalation and upper airway burns may precipitate airway edema and obstruction within 24–48 hours after the burn.

- Inhalation of carbon monoxide combines with hemoglobin, thereby decreasing oxygen availability to cells.

Important nursing implications	Serious/life-threatening implications
Most frequent side effects	Patient teaching

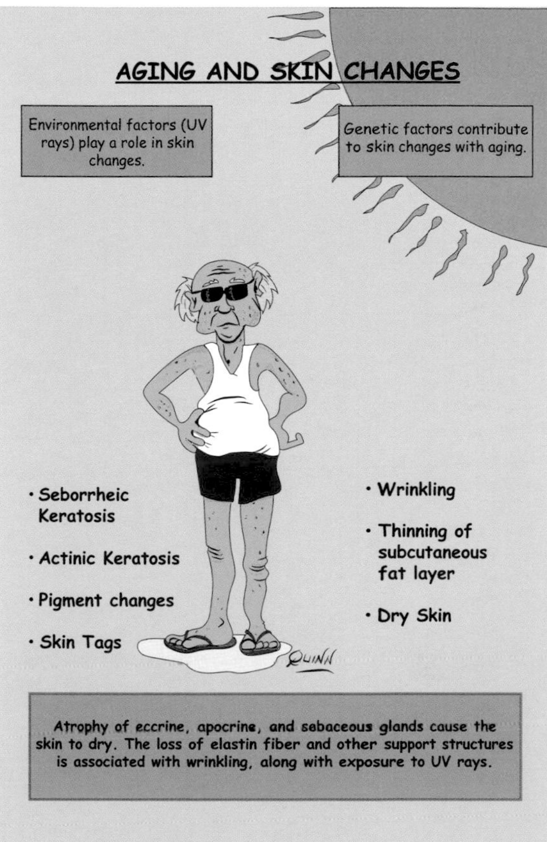
AGING AND SKIN CHANGES
Environmental factors (UV rays) play a role in skin changes.
Genetic factors contribute to skin changes with aging.
• Seborrheic Keratosis
• Actinic Keratosis
• Pigment changes
• Skin Tags
• Wrinkling
• Thinning of subcutaneous fat layer
• Dry Skin
QUINN
Atrophy of eccrine, apocrine, and sebaceous glands cause the skin to dry. The loss of elastin fiber and other support structures is associated with wrinkling, along with exposure to UV rays.

What You Need to Know

Aging and Skin Changes

SIGNIFICANCE OF AGE-RELATED SKIN CHANGES

Age-related skin changes are influenced by heredity, personal history of sun exposure, hygiene practices, nutrition, and general state of health.

- Although the number of cell layers remains unchanged, the epidermis thins.
- Melanocytes decrease in number, but the remaining melanocytes increase in size, leaving the skin thin, pale, and translucent. The hair begins to turn gray.
- Large, pigmented spots (called *age spots*, *liver spots*, or *lentigos*) may appear in sun-exposed areas.
- Seborrheic keratosis, noncancerous skin lesions, appear more in the gerontology population. The lesion usually appears as brown wartlike growth on the head, neck, chest, or back.
- Actinic keratosis is a precancerous lesion that appears as a rough, scaly patch seen in areas of the body that are exposed to sun (face, lips, ears, forearms, and scalp).
- Changes in the connective tissue reduce the skin's strength and elastioity, causing wrinkling. The loss of skin elasticity produces the leathery, weather-beaten appearance common to farmers, sailors, and others who spend a large amount of time outdoors, as well as smokers.
- Blood vessels of the dermis become more fragile, which leads to bruising, bleeding under the skin, spider angiomas, and similar conditions.
- Sebaceous glands produce less oil. Men experience a minimal decrease, usually after the age of 80 years. Women gradually produce less oil, beginning after menopause, which leads to dry and itchy skin.
- Thinning of the subcutaneous fat layer increases the risk of skin injury and reduces the ability to maintain body temperature, which leads to increased risk of hypothermia.
- Eccrine and apocrine sweat glands atrophy, leading to dry skin and decreased body odor.
- Smokers tend to have more wrinkles than nonsmokers of the same age, complexion, and history of sun exposure.

NURSING IMPLICATIONS

- Educate individuals on the importance of using sunscreen products, with spf 30 or higher, to reduce the effects of photoaging—wrinkling, solar lentigos, and actinic keratosis.
- Annual skin assessment should be done to evaluate for changes in skin lesions.

Important nursing implications | Serious/life-threatening implications
Most frequent side effects | Patient teaching

Index

Page numbers followed by *f* indicate figures and *t* indicate tables.

C

D

E

J

K

L

M

N

R

S

T